10-DAY SUGAR DETOX

Ready to Detox?

Prepare for lifestyle changes. See page 16.

Learn where sugar hides. See page 19.

Decide which detox plan is right for you. See page 31.

Create a detox-friendly kitchen. See page 51.

Eat sugar-free. Recipes start on page 70

● ● ● ●

10-DAY SUGAR DETOX

EASY MEAL PLANS TO BEAT SUGAR IN 10 DAYS

Foreword by **DANA ANGELO WHITE, MS, RD**

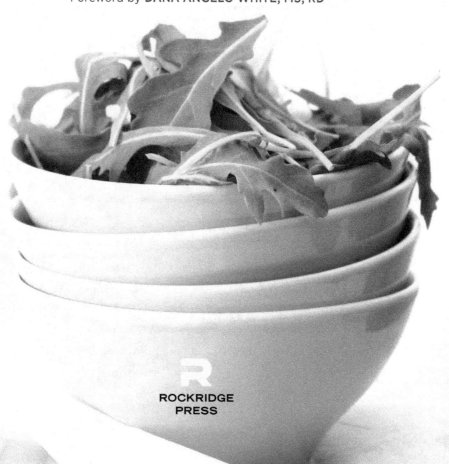

ROCKRIDGE
PRESS

For general information on our other products and services or to obtain technical support, please contact our Customer Care Department within the United States at (866) 744-2665, or outside the United States at (510) 253-0500.

Rockridge Press publishes its books in a variety of electronic and print formats. Some content that appears in print may not be available in electronic books, and vice versa.

PHOTO CREDITS: Shutterstock/Torok-Bognar Renata, p.3; Shutterstock/Jill Chen, p.8; Stockfood/ Holly Pickering, p.11; StockFood/Greg Rannells Photography, p.12; StockFood/Keller & Keller Photography, p.20; StockFood/Westend61, p.29; Shutterstock/Olha Afanasieva, p.30; Shutterstock/ B. and E. Dudzinscy, p.50; Sarka Babicka, p.60; StockFood/Sarka Babicka, p.67; StockFood/Brigitte Sporrer, p.68; StockFood/ISTL, p.90; StockFood/Rua Castilho, p.106; StockFood/Linda Pugliese, p.126; StockFood/Gräfe & Unzer Verlag/Rynio, Jörn, p.154; Stockfood/Stuart West, p.172; StockFood/Rose Hodges, p.190; StockFood/Marc O. Finley, p.204; Shutterstock/B. and E. Dudzinscy, p.218

ISBN: Print 978-1-62315-426-4 | eBook 978-1-62315-427-1

CONTENTS

Foreword by Dana Angelo White, MS, RD 6
Introduction 9

Part I: The Sugar Detox Solution
One Are You Ready to Quit Sugar? *12*
Two Sugar and How It Works *20*

Part II: Your 10-Day Detox
Three Choosing Your Detox and Planning for It *30*
Four Preparing for Your Detox *50*
Five After the Detox *60*

Part III: 10-Day Sugar Detox Recipes
Six Breakfast *68*
Seven Make-Ahead Snacks *90*
Eight Salads, Soups, Sandwiches & Sides *106*
Nine Vegetarian Mains *126*
Ten Seafood & Fish *154*
Eleven Poultry & Meat *172*
Twelve After-Dinner Treats *190*
Thirteen Condiments, Dressings & Sauces *204*

Appendix A: Resources 219
Appendix B: Measurement Conversions 221
References 222
Recipe Index 225
Index 227

FOREWORD

As a nutrition professional, my job is to help people understand how to eat better so that they can feel better—and often look better, too. Some of my clients think they know what they want from me: plans to reduce the amount of cholesterol in their diets, recipes to make whole-foods meals quickly, and/or advice for how to balance work, eating, and exercise. Few people come to me ready to acknowledge, or even aware, that they have a problem with their sugar intake. Having worked with everyone from regular folks to hardcore athletes, I know that sugar overconsumption is a problem that most of us can't afford to ignore.

In 2013 the Centers for Disease Control and Prevention released data noting that Americans take in as much as 16 percent of their total calories from added sugars. All of this extra sugar contributes to a staggering amount of empty calories gobbled up, which stresses the metabolism and can lead to obesity and other health problems.

But when it comes to cutting out sugar, it is not as simple as making one small change to your diet; if it were that easy, a lot more people would do it. The biggest challenge many of my patients face when they attempt to cut back on sugar is that they often underestimate its prevalence in what they eat. Sugar is lurking in so many unexpected foods and beverages. Candy and soda are clearly sugar-laden fare, but jarred marinara sauce, bottled salad dressings, and even marinades are less obvious offenders.

The 10-Day Sugar Detox offered in this book is designed to clear from your diet processed foods and other less-than-healthy ingredients in a sensible, satisfying, and—most importantly—safe manner. Fresh, whole-food ingredients are featured in recipes filled with complex flavors that are also incredibly simple to make. I especially like the option of following one of several color-coded plans, because they are designed to accommodate just about everyone. Whether you have to avoid gluten or choose to follow a vegetarian diet, there's a plan that can fit your lifestyle.

Now, I do need to confess something. As a health care professional, how the word "detox" is used today leaves me a little unsettled. There are just too many detox plans that promise to rid your body of harmful substances while requiring starvation, the exclusion of entire food groups, the use of dangerous supplements, and other potentially risky tactics. There are plenty of good reasons to be wary of fad detox plans, and you should give serious thought to any detox before undertaking it. This book aims to offer a very basic education about sugar and then provides recipes for simple, healthy, no-sugar meals. Many of my clients have benefited from cutting sugar out of their diets from time to time. This book is here to help you do it, too.

A plan can get you started, but the work of implementing it is up to you. Do your best to stick to it, and enjoy the increased energy and more balanced eating it brings over the next 10 days—or longer.

Dana Angelo White, MS, RD
September 2014

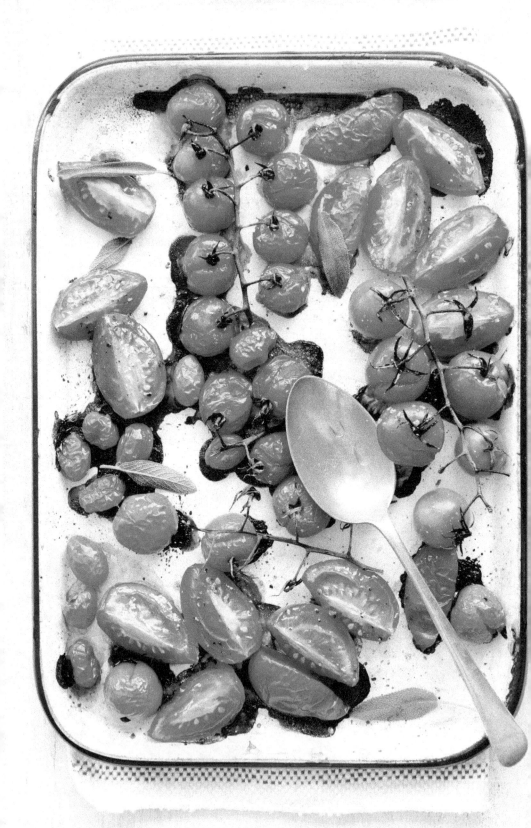

INTRODUCTION

Mary Poppins famously sang that "a spoonful of sugar helps the medicine go down." But what about the five teaspoons mixed into your so-called healthy, low-fat yogurt?

With hidden sugars lurking in just about every food available on the market—from condiments to breakfast cereals to canned fruits and almost anything labeled "fat-free"—America has become a nation of unintentional sugar addicts. According to the United States Department of Agriculture, each year Americans consume an average of 142 pounds of added sugar per person, and many studies have linked this high intake of added sugar to serious conditions such as obesity, type 2 diabetes, and heart disease. Other recognized side effects of high added-sugar intake include lack of energy and focus, trouble sleeping, and digestive issues.

Though it may seem extreme to banish all sugars from your diet at once, a temporary detox can help you reboot your system and free yourself from dependency. Removing sugar from your diet for the short term may help you live a fuller, longer life.

In this book you will learn about the devastating impact sugar has on your health, and how removing it from your system for just 10 days can detoxify your body and get you on the right path to long-term well being.

10-Day Sugar Detox can help you kick your sugar habits with four different 10-day detox plans that meet you where you are and take you where you want to be. Make no mistake: These detoxes are restrictive and require a firm commitment, but they're also highly structured, sensible, and intended to free you from your sugar addiction. In the process, they assist in the removal of toxins, establish smart eating habits, and jump-start your body's healing process.

The four detoxes each come with a 10-day meal plan to ensure that you cut out all refined sugars over a 10-day period. One of the detoxes even offers all-vegetarian meals for those interested in going both sugar-free and meat-free.

Whether you're looking to lose weight and keep it off, build better eating habits, live cleaner and longer, stave off disease, or do any combination of these, *10-Day Sugar Detox* can be your meal ticket to a healthier life.

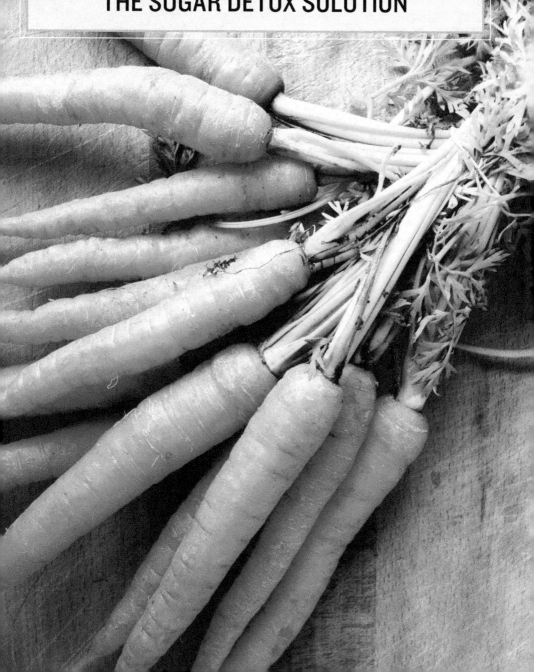

PART I

THE SUGAR DETOX SOLUTION

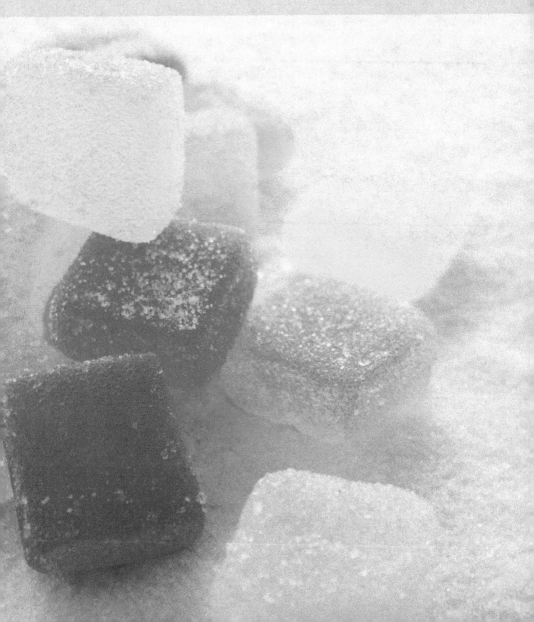

ONE

ARE YOU READY TO QUIT SUGAR?

An innocent spread of jam across your toast, that late-afternoon pick-me-up soda, even a ladle of your dinner pasta sauce . . . they all contain some sugar. The amounts may seem small and insignificant by themselves, but they add up in a big way. Day after day, month after month, you consume much more sugar than you realize, and over time that can lead to serious problems such as obesity, heart disease, and type 2 diabetes, not to mention feelings of fatigue, inability to focus, and indigestion.

As this book shows, these everyday food choices can be the root cause of many of your health and wellness issues. But in order to break your addiction and free yourself from excess sugar, you have to be ready to quit. Only then can you begin to detoxify your body so it can heal itself.

A Healthier Lifestyle Begins Now

As the saying goes, you're bound to lose every race you don't enter. So if you want to feel more energetic, lose weight, sleep better, think more clearly, and live longer, then you have to change your lifestyle.

But how do you begin? And what comes afterward? If you're reading this book, you've already made a great first step toward booting added sugars from your diet and reaping the health benefits that will inevitably follow. Now you just need to learn the ins and outs of the plan, and you'll be well on your way to a healthier mind and body.

The 10-Day Sugar Detox plan is easy to follow, requires only a short time commitment, and can even be customized to your individual tastes, dietary restrictions, and budget. In this book you will find four different color-coded meal plans to choose from, all of which are free of gluten. While other sugar detox plans serve up the same item day after day for regular meals—e.g., a protein shake for breakfast—here you are offered choices to keep your meals flavorful and varied.

By following one of the four detox plans outlined here, you can break your sugar dependency once and for all, cleanse your body, restart your sluggish metabolism, and get your health moving in the right direction. In the span of your life, a 10-day period barely registers, yet if you stick with the sugar detox plan outlined in this book, you'll find even that short period of time can make a big difference. It won't always be easy, but after just 10 days you can free your body of refined sugar and create better dietary habits that can last a lifetime.

Reasons to Do a 10-Day Detox

The 10-Day Sugar Detox is your blueprint for building a new outlook on what and how to eat. It's not a quick fix or one-time solution. It's not something that must be repeated every few months to work. It's a strategy to teach you better eating habits and cleanse your body so you can grow healthier. In just 10 days you can begin to feel the various wonderful effects of a life less dependent on sugar. Here are a few of the results you can expect from the plans offered here:

WEIGHT LOSS. Research has shown that eating more sugar is tied to weight gain and eating less sugar is linked to weight loss. For example, one national literature review in the *American Journal of Clinical Nutrition* noted an association between intake of sugar-sweetened beverages such as soda and weight gain. If you want to stop the yo-yo dieting, lose those extra pounds, and keep them off, then you need to detoxify your body from sugar.

BETTER EATING HABITS. When you're able to overcome your sugar addiction, you replace those sugary foods with healthy choices. You'll eat more whole fruits and vegetables, vitamin-packed greens, lean meats, wholesome grains, and "good" fats. No more processed and packaged items. No more eating out of a box. Without the overload of sugar, you'll realize that real food does not have to be *created*. It already exists in its pure, natural form and provides all the nutrients you need to cleanse and nourish your body.

BETTER SLEEP. According to data obtained from an assessment tool called the National Health Interview Survey, almost 30 percent of adults get less than six hours of sleep per night on average, which is far below the seven to eight hours most experts recommend. Excess sugar may be the reason you have trouble falling asleep or keep waking up during the night. Longtime sugar addiction can lead to anxiety and depression, and both conditions are known to disrupt sleep patterns. And since sugar is an energy source, you may often

What Is a Detox?

Detox is short for *detoxification*, which is a natural, ongoing process. Every second of every day, your body is detoxifying itself. Your skin, kidneys, liver, intestines, and lymphatic system all work alone and together to purify your body by neutralizing and/or eliminating toxins. Toxins are anything that can cause potential harm, whether they come from the environment, food, or other exposure.

Every day people ingest or are exposed to chemicals, which can get deposited in the body's fat cells. A 2009 data review published in the *International Journal of Environmental Research and Public Health* showed that some of these toxins may serve as endocrine disrupters, which can lead to weight gain.

Detox diets are dietary plans designed to help support your detox system as well as remove toxins and protect the body from future invaders. The philosophy is that by eliminating specific foods and emphasizing others, you can heal the body and boost the performance of your natural detox system.

reach for sugary foods and drinks to fuel your sluggish mornings. Breaking your sugar habit can reset your sleeping patterns and help you get the slumber you need for a healthy body and brain.

HEALTHY DIGESTION. The National Institute of Diabetes and Digestive and Kidney Diseases notes that certain sugars, like lactose, may cause digestive issues in intolerant individuals. These sugars often trigger digestive issues like gas, bloating, cramps, and diarrhea. Take out the sugar, though, and you can begin to repair your digestive tract and end stomach problems. Also, when you remove sugar from your diet, you avoid consuming sugar-laden processed foods. These foods are often broken down into molecules that your body senses as toxic and fires a surge of antibodies to fight. If you depend on processed foods, you put your body on autopilot to wage a constant attack.

What to Expect During the 10-Day Detox

Lasting change, such as cutting down on added sugar in your diet, demands commitment and dedication in order to be successful. The 10-Day Sugar Detox plan can help you create the change you desire, but you have to be prepared to face some challenges along the way.

Higher Grocery Bills

You're about to become more mindful of what you eat, how much, and how often. When you hit the grocery store to shop for this detox, you'll be purchasing whole foods; fresh and sometimes organic produce, herbs, and spices; and other ingredients that might be entirely new to you. They are absolutely healthier than what you have been eating, but odds are they'll cost more too. Don't let that discourage you. A sugarless diet is not inherently an expensive one. The initial cost spike is because a change such as this requires starting anew with what you buy. If your diet consists of a fair number of packaged and frozen foods, and if your pantry is relatively low on herbs, spices, and healthy cooking oils, it might feel like you're stocking a kitchen from scratch. If you are used to cooking "whole foods" on a regular basis but simply want a rigorous program to get sugar out of your diet once and for all, you might find that you don't have to buy many new pantry items at all.

Keep in mind that you'll get use out of pantry staples, such as flours and oils, over and over again. You will need to replenish the fresh foods more often, of course, but take heart in knowing that you'll be eating the very best that nature has to offer. You are investing in your health for today and tomorrow. Every extra dollar you spend now can keep you from potentially costly medical issues down the road.

More Time Spent in the Kitchen

Whether you love to cook or are a complete novice, you will become more kitchen savvy following this 10-day detox. Because you'll be more involved with your eating—from shopping to cooking—this is a wonderful opportunity to embrace your culinary skills and take charge of your meal preparation. But the best part is that the four meal plans offered here are designed to be low-maintenance with easy-to-follow instructions. If the kitchen is an unfamiliar place, keep in mind that you may have to adjust your mind-set and schedule to accommodate your new eating lifestyle. You may have to prep parts of meals beforehand and give yourself the extra time to cook until you find your groove. You only have to be this new kind of chef for 10 days, but you may find yourself referencing the techniques and recipes in this book long after you've completed your detox.

Regular Exercise Requirements

Changing your diet is only part of the equation. You also have to incorporate some kind of physical activity. As your body and its systems begin to adjust to the detoxification process, exercise becomes vital. A regular exercise routine consisting of at least 30 minutes per day can fuel your body and brain as well as fight off cravings for sugar during the 10-day plan and beyond. When you don't exercise, you're more likely to crave sugary foods for comfort, especially when faced with stress. It doesn't matter what you do, as long as you commit to something. Run or jog, take a Zumba class, do yoga, go for a walk, ride your bike, or swim. Focus on what you enjoy, and go from there. But get moving.

Sugar Withdrawal

Your body is used to sugar. It expects it and depends on it. So now that you'll suddenly be removing it and depriving your system of what it craves, you'll experience some form of withdrawal. You should also be aware that replacing sugary junk with high-fiber, whole foods can also cause some initial digestive distress. It's natural but short-term. For the first couple of days the symptoms may vary in frequency and severity, often including uncomfortable sensations like nausea, fatigue, headaches, irritability, anxiety, and moodiness. But this is a good thing, as it signals that your body is detoxing and beginning to heal. As your system gets less accustomed to relying on sugar, it will adjust and begin to work at more optimal levels. See chapter 3 for more information on preparing your body for a sugar detox and dealing with withdrawal symptoms as they arise.

You Can Do It

One of the advantages of this sugar detox is its duration. It lasts for only 10 days and is therefore far less intimidating than other plans that stretch over 21 days, 8 weeks, or even longer. And since your initial obligation is so brief, there is little opportunity to lose focus or excitement.

It's tough to find any other kind of lifestyle strategy that can institute such lasting behavior in such a short period. You cannot begin a workout plan and expect huge results in only 10 days. Nor can you lose a significant amount of weight on a 10-day diet without embracing drastic, potentially dangerous eating habits.

But in only 10 days, the sugar detox can break your sugar addiction and help you learn new eating and lifestyle habits that can accelerate your life in a new direction. You will eat smarter and more healthily and feel better and stronger. Everyone has 10 days they can devote to making such fundamental changes.

Consulting a Doctor

It's essential that you consult with your physician before undertaking any kind of nutritional plan or diet, but especially if you have any type of medical condition or are taking prescription medication. Any sudden change in your diet, as with the 10-Day Sugar Detox, may affect how medication interacts in your system. Even if you're in ideal health with no major medical issues, your doctor should be aware of your intentions and goals in order to provide necessary advice and guidance. Depending on your age, gender, and medical background, you may need to adjust the recipe strategy here to meet your individual needs.

Sugar by Any Other Name

Sugar goes by many different names. The obvious ones have *sugar*, *juice*, or *syrup* as part of their names or end with "ose," like *fructose*, *sucrose*, *dextrose*, *saccharose*, and *maltose*. Others, especially artificial sweeteners, sugar substitutes, and sugar alcohols, sound like they belong in a lab. Scan food labels for any of these names, and be sure to avoid them during your sugar detox:

- Acesulfame potassium
- Agave nectar
- Aspartame
- Cyclamate
- Dextrin
- Diatase ·
- Erythritol
- Ethyl maltol
- Fructamyl
- Glycerol
- Glycyrrhizin
- Hydrogenated starch hydrolysate
- Isomalt
- Lactitol
- Maltitol
- Maltodextrin
- Mannitol
- Neotame
- Panocha
- Polydextrose
- Saccharin
- Sorbitol
- Sucralose
- Tagatose
- Treacle
- Xylitol

TWO

SUGAR AND HOW IT WORKS

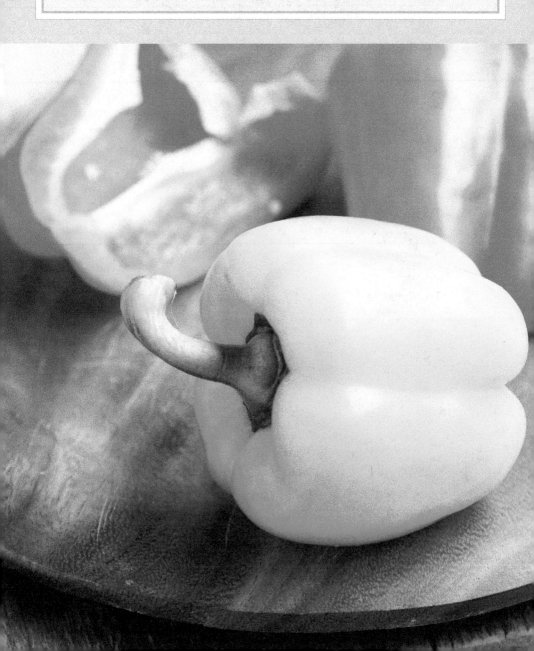

Before you shake off sugar, you need to know what it is and how it works. First of all, it's important to note that sugar itself is not "evil." In fact, your body relies on glucose—or simple sugars—for energy.

Carbohydrates and Sugar

During the digestive process, the carbohydrates found in food are broken down into single glucose molecules that are then released into the blood to fuel cells with energy. The three types of carbohydrates that are converted to glucose in the body are starch, fiber, and sugar, and each type breaks down differently according to its molecular makeup.

Starch and fiber are complex carbohydrates, sometimes referred to as "good" carbs. They can be made up of hundreds of molecules of sugar and therefore take longer to digest, resulting in a slow, steady introduction of glucose to the bloodstream.

Sugar is a simple carbohydrate and has been labeled a "bad" carb because its components break down very quickly, which makes them more likely to cause spikes in blood sugar. Sucrose is the simple sugar (think of table sugar) that we tend to add in cooking, but some whole foods naturally contain simple sugars, too—for example, fructose in fruit and lactose in milk are simple sugars. Because whole foods offer many benefits to the body, it's shortsighted to dismiss them from the diet on the sole basis that they contain simple sugars.

Natural and Refined Sugars

Where your body gets sugar from makes a huge difference. The easiest way to look at sugar is to split it into two groups: natural and refined.

NATURAL SUGAR. Found in whole foods like fruits and milk, natural sugar (as previously mentioned) is also in vegetables, beans, nuts, and whole grains. Though in its simplest state it has the same makeup as refined sugar, natural sugar also comes with good stuff like disease-fighting antioxidants, phytonutrients, essential vitamins and minerals, and fiber. The presence of fiber makes a significant difference because it slows down the absorption of sugar, which moderates its impact on your blood sugar levels. Fiber also expands in your gut, making you feel full so you're less likely to overconsume.

That said, not all natural sugar foods are the same. Some fruits, such as cherries and grapes, contain particularly high amounts of natural sugar. These are delicious, wholesome fruits that have a place in a regular diet, but their sugar content is higher than appropriate for a detox. Lemons, limes, and some berries (such as blueberries and blackberries) have very low levels of sugar, so they are allowed in small quantities on the detox. They won't get you craving sugar. To help break your addiction and curb your dependency on sugar, you have to keep blood sugar levels in check, and these sources of natural sugar do that while providing your body with other vital nutrients.

Although fruit is beneficial to your health, it is the most powerful in its natural whole state. Once fruit has been altered in any way through cooking or juicing, its nutritional benefits decline and its fiber becomes less constructed. So while that morning glass of orange juice is still rich in nutrients, its much higher concentration of sugar and much lower amounts of fiber make it an unwise choice for the detox plan. This is also true for all other fruit food, such as applesauce and jams.

REFINED SUGAR. A refined sugar is one that is added to foods during processing, used in cooking and baking, stirred into coffee or tea, or sprinkled on cereal. The problems with refined sugar are its fast rate of metabolism, lack of healthy nutrients, and inability to make you feel full. Refined sugar is quickly broken down into glucose. The increase in glucose spikes insulin and blood sugar levels, giving you a quick surge of energy. If you don't use this energy immediately, your body can turn it into fat. And because it lacks fiber, refined sugar gets digested quickly and doesn't give your brain time to register that you've had enough, so you may eat more and more sugar to satisfy your hunger.

Sugar Overload

We've established that your body turns extra glucose into fat, but it's worth understanding the process a bit more, as well as why high fat storage is more than just a cosmetic problem.

When there is an excess of glucose in the bloodstream, the liver converts some of it into fatty acids—that is, fat—and deposits it back

Is Detox Possible While Eating Natural Sugars?

The short answer is yes. Again, sugar is not an evil substance. It has a role in your overall health and wellness. But for the 10-Day Sugar Detox, you want to break that dependency on sugar and cut out the sweet cravings. Though you will refrain from most refined sugar sources while on the detox, certain natural sugars—the kinds found in fruits and dairy—are allowed in moderation. They supply essential nutrients as well as fiber to help control appetite and provide feelings of satisfaction.

into the bloodstream. Here it tours your body and then gets stored away. Common fat deposit areas include the stomach, hips, butt, and breasts. When your body stores too much fat, health problems can develop such as high blood pressure, low metabolism, and a weakened immune system. Some of that glucose in the bloodstream also gets converted to low-density lipoprotein, more commonly known as LDL or "bad" cholesterol, which can form plaque in blood vessels and increase your risk of heart attack.

The Role of Insulin

When sugar intake balloons, so, too, does the body's production of insulin. Insulin has a very specific job: to regulate the amount of glucose in the blood. Whenever you consume foods that are broken down into glucose, insulin is released into your bloodstream and distributed to cells throughout the body. The insulin attaches itself to individual cells and allows the glucose to move from the blood into the cell, where it is converted to energy. When you consume large amounts of sugar, sending a flood of glucose into the bloodstream, the body reacts with a spike in insulin. If these spikes become a regular occurrence, they compromise the body's ability to properly control blood sugar—and may lead to metabolic problems, including an increased risk for type 2 diabetes.

Any remaining glucose travels into your liver, as mentioned earlier, and muscles. When your muscles reach their sugar capacity, your body also slows its insulin production. Blood sugar levels fall. Your appetite increases, which makes you crave more food—often the sugary kind— and the stress hormone cortisol is activated. Cortisol triggers the release of stored glucose from the liver, which, combined with the extra food you probably ate thanks to your new appetite, begins the entire sugar-overload/fat-storage process again. According to *Today's Dietitian*, a magazine written for nutrition professionals, when cortisol is "chronically elevated," or too high over an extended period of time, it can harm the healthy operation of the immune system, increase the risk of chronic disease, and negatively affect weight.

Sugar Addiction

With the list of nasty side effects growing by the day, there seem to be more and more reasons to banish added sugars from our diets— and yet processed foods and sugary soft drinks show no signs of disappearing from grocery store shelves nationwide. The problem? It seems that the more sugar you eat, the more sugar you crave.

There's a reason why experts call it a sugar addiction. In many ways your dependence on sweets is similar to drug use. In 2008, research led by Bart Hoebel, PhD, at the Princeton Neuroscience Institute found that intermittent sugar intake in rats caused changes in the animals' brains and behavior similar to those from drugs such as cocaine, morphine, and nicotine. In Hoebel's studies, the animals also experienced withdrawal symptoms when their sugar was taken away, such as anxiety, isolation, and intense cravings.

When you consume sugar, your brain releases a surge of the neurotransmitter dopamine, also known as the "feel-good hormone." It makes you feel content and relaxed, which is why that slice of cake or cold soda is so pleasing, especially when you are stressed. It doesn't just taste good—it feels good, too. And especially for those prone to addiction, it can be a very hard habit to break.

Beyond Cookies and Cake: Six Foods to Limit or Exclude

Some sources of sugar are easy to target for elimination—for example, cookies, cake, candy, and junk food like snack and processed foods.

But there are also foods you don't associate with high sugar that are equally important to stay away from during your 10-day detox. The following six items are excluded or restricted in the 10-Day Sugar Detox's four meal plans as they contain either high amounts of sugar or simple ("bad") carbohydrates. These foods may offer specific nutritional qualities, but for this sugar detox you want to limit their role in your diet.

1. **Gluten.** *Not allowed.* Gluten is a combination of two proteins, gliadin and glutenin, found in wheat, barley, and rye. It is ground into flour that is then used to make bread, pizza, cereal, pasta, pastries, crackers, and cookies. Gluten is what gives these foods their doughy elasticity and chewy texture. It is also added to foods like processed soups, salad dressings, and condiments and drinks such as beer. Gluten-free diets are not optional for people with celiac disease, who have trouble digesting gluten, or for those with gluten sensitivities. But numerous foods containing gluten are also sources of simple carbohydrates.

2. **Caffeine.** *Not allowed.* The elimination of caffeine has several purposes in a sugar detox. It helps you resist the temptation to add sugar to your morning coffee or tea, and it helps cut out sugary beverages like soda and sports drinks. Caffeine is also a stimulant and reacts in the body much like sugar. If you want to detoxify your body and break your dependency on sugar, you want to avoid anything that might replicate the effects of sugar. This allows your body and brain to reset from the constant bombardment of stimulation.

3. **Grains.** *Allowed on some meal plans.* Grains are carbohydrates, and as this chapter has shown, carbs get converted into sugar in the body. They're good in that they offer high nutritional quality and also provide a quick energy source, which is why they're popular for pre- and post-workout meals and snacks. But since carbs are digested quickly in the body, it takes longer for your brain to register when you are full, and this can lead to over-eating. Since the 10-Day Sugar Detox helps you better manage your blood sugar, you want to be careful with foods that can

cause sudden spikes. Grains aren't on the "no" list for all detox plans, but they are used sparingly.

4. **Legumes.** *Allowed on some meal plans.* Legumes have a similar story to grains. They're a great protein source, especially if you are a vegetarian or limit your intake of meat. They may also help prevent the onset of type 2 diabetes, notes a 2008 study in the *American Journal of Clinical Nutrition*. The study showed that legume consumption was inversely correlated with development of the condition. Yet, a major drawback of legumes is their lectin content. Lectins are sticky, carb-binding proteins that can attach to the intestinal lining and, according to the *British Medical Journal*, can have an inflammatory effect on the digestive system. While some people have no reaction to lectins, those who do can follow the detoxes that do not contain legumes without worry.

5. **Dairy.** *Allowed on some meal plans.* Dairy is allowed on some of the plans—for vegetarians, for whom it can provide an importance source of calcium and protein, and for those easing into a sugar detox for the first time. It is not allowed on the more restrictive detox plans because meat provides the necessary protein, and because those inclined to be very strict about detoxing may not want even the natural sugar (lactose) found in dairy.

Regardless of the plan you undertake, you may wish to consider giving up dairy for the 10-day period. Dairy products like milk, yogurt, and ice cream contain high amounts of the sugar lactose. Many adults have lactose intolerance, a condition that impedes the body's digestion of lactose and results in uncomfortable symptoms such as bloating and gas. This can interfere with digestion and cause extra stress. In fact, WebMD estimates that between 30 and 50 million Americans have some degree of lactose intolerance.

Some people may tolerate dairy poorly for additional reasons as well. According to the Mayo Clinic, both of milk's primary proteins, casein and whey, may cause allergic reactions in sensitive individuals. Food Allergy Research and

Fruit and Dairy Allowed Per Day

For those following detoxes that allow fruit and dairy, keep in mind that these meal plans are limited to no more than **2 servings** of each per day. Here's a guide to what 1 serving entails:

- 1 serving fruit = 1 cup or 1 piece

- 1 serving dairy = 1 cup milk or yogurt, ⅓ cup shredded cheese, 1.5 ounces hard cheese, or ½ cup ricotta cheese

Education (FARE) notes that about 2.5 percent of children under the age of three have milk allergies. Reactions can range from mild inflammation to life-threatening anaphylaxis.

6. **Fruit.** *Allowed but restricted.* Fruit is not eliminated on the 10-Day Sugar Detox, but it's limited to a very small number of fruits across all four meal plans: avocados, green-tipped bananas, blackberries, blueberries, lemons, limes, strawberries, and tomatoes. While fruit boasts many nutritional benefits, especially fiber, it can also have high levels of the natural sugar fructose. Though the health benefits of fruit are indisputable, to fully detoxify your body from sugar, you have to block out the major everyday sources. And fruit can feed your body a steady supply of sugar, whether it is whole, frozen, juiced, dried, or canned (with added juice).

Zero/Low Calorie and Sugar-Free Foods

These foods may sound better for you than others, but that doesn't mean they're not packed with added sugars. Here's a look behind these misleading labels.

Zero/Low Calorie. Sodas and foods labeled with low or no calories sound like they're good for you, but what they lack in calories they make up for in sugar and additives. They often contain artificial sweeteners and sugar alcohols. Research in *Obesity Reviews* finds that consuming large amounts of these food products can interfere with the natural bacteria in your intestines, which slows your metabolism and disrupts the body's way of signaling that you are full and satisfied.

Sugar-Free. "No sugar" does not mean an absence of sweeteners. "Sugar-free" means that a product contains less than 0.5 grams of sugars per serving, according to the Food and Drug Administration. However, companies can make a sugar-free claim by also using artificial sweeteners or sugar alcohols. Most foods that contain artificial sweeteners are highly processed and offer little in terms of nutrition.

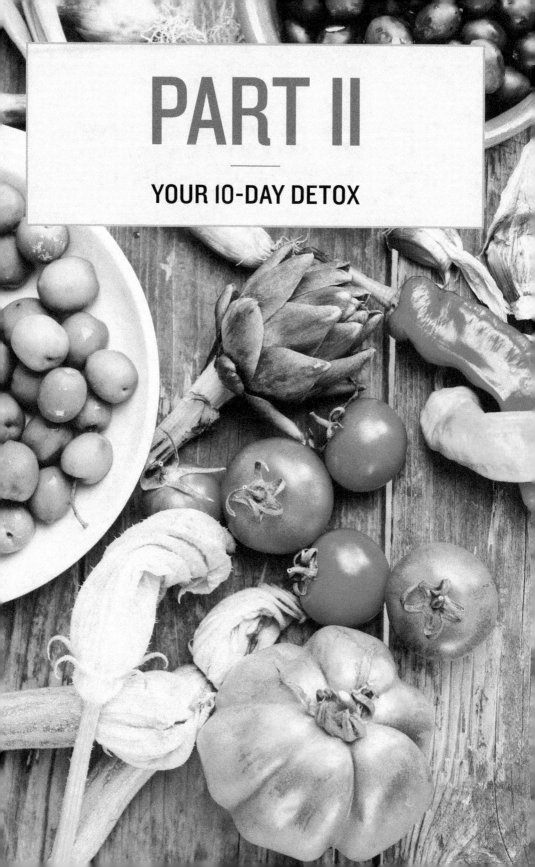

PART II

YOUR 10-DAY DETOX

THREE

CHOOSING YOUR DETOX AND PLANNING FOR IT

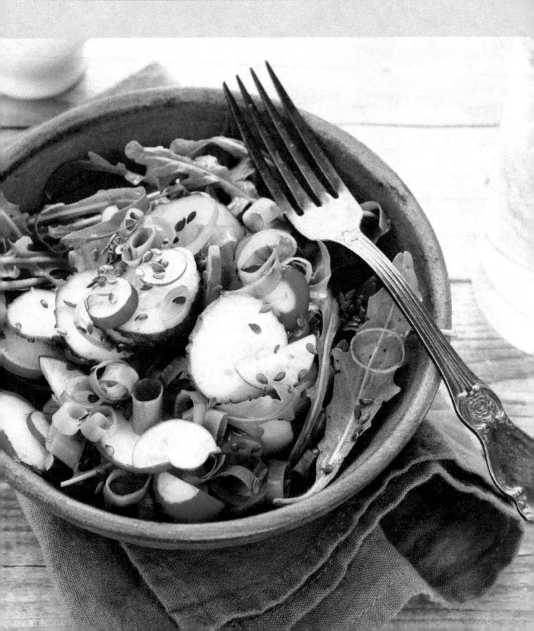

In this section, you'll find four different 10-Day Sugar Detox meal plans to suit your individual needs. The plans range according to restrictions, from allowing both full-fat dairy and gluten-free grains to excluding both. Under the heading for each meal plan, you'll find a brief description of the foods included and excluded from that plan, a schedule of meals to eat during your 10-day detox, and a detailed shopping list. Each meal plan includes 10 days' worth of breakfasts, snacks, lunches, and dinners. Simply prepare and enjoy the suggested meal at the designated time each day for the entire 10-day meal plan.

During a sugar detox, it's likely that you'll be especially aware of your sweet tooth. The meal plans provided here do not include a traditional dessert, of course. But in chapter 12, you'll find a handful of recipes for after-dinner treats that serve up sweet or savory bites, with no added sugars. When you're tempted to cheat, turn to this chapter. You won't be cheating, but it just might feel like you are.

Which Detox Is Right for You?

One of the most valuable features of this sugar detox cookbook is that there isn't only one detox that everyone has to do. People detox for various reasons and have different health concerns, habits, and motivations. You can select a detox plan that accommodates your individual nutritional needs and preferences. In order to help you make the right choice, refer to the four color-coded profiles below, which provide examples of the lifestyle and dietary preferences of the followers of each plan.

Each of these meal plans limits fruit to two serving per day, and none of them allows beverages such as alcohol, fruit juice, or soft drinks.

● *Orange Plan*

The Orange meal plan excludes poultry, fish, and meat. This plan includes limited full-fat dairy products and gluten-free grains and legumes to ensure that those eating vegetarian for the duration of the detox consume enough fat and protein. Dairy is limited to one serving (see chapter 2, page 26 for specific serving information).

This plan is recommended for individuals who:

- Have never completed a sugar detox before
- Have been following a vegetarian diet or are interested in following a vegetarian diet for a short period of time
- Have no known food allergies or intolerances
- Have made few to no significant changes to their recent dietary habits

Yellow Plan

The Yellow meal plan is the least restrictive of the four plans, but you shouldn't interpret that to mean that it is the easiest. This plan includes meat as well as limited full-fat dairy products, gluten-free grains, and legumes. Dairy is limited to one serving (see chapter 2, page 26 for specific serving information).

This plan is recommended for individuals who:

- Have never completed a sugar detox before
- Have few dietary restrictions or have never made significant dietary changes before
- Have no known food allergies or intolerances
- Have made few to no significant changes to their recent dietary habits

Green Plan

The Green meal plan is moderately restrictive in the sense that it includes meat and full-fat dairy but excludes grains (even gluten-free grains) and legumes. Dairy is limited to one serving (see chapter 2, page 26 for specific serving information).

This plan is recommended for individuals who:

- Are familiar with detoxing and may have tried a detox before
- Have some experience with making conscious changes to their diet
- Prefer not to eat gluten (or are medically restricted from doing so)
- Are familiar or have experience with the Paleo diet or similar diets

A Word on Supplements

Many detoxification plans advocate the use of supplements—
either individual vitamins and minerals or multivitamins and
vitamin formulas—to ensure that your body gets the nutritional
support it needs. Food is always the best option. For the 10-Day
Sugar Detox, no supplements are required; if you follow the meal
plans provided in this book, your body will have all the nutrients it
needs during the detoxification process.

● *Blue Plan*

The Blue meal plan is the most restrictive of the four plans, but it
should not be interpreted as the most difficult plan; if this meal plan
is right for you, you have already given serious thought to restricting
various foods from your diet. This plan includes meat but excludes
all dairy, grains, and legumes.

This plan is recommended for individuals who:

- Are familiar with detoxing and/or have successfully
  completed a detox

- Have made significant conscious changes to their dietary
  habits in the past

- Have food allergies or intolerances (especially to wheat,
  gluten, or dairy)

- Have experience with the Paleo diet or similar diets

● ORANGE PLAN

When following the Orange meal plan, you will consume eggs and dairy, vegetables, nuts and seeds, and gluten-free grains and legumes. This meal plan also includes soy products and is ideal for those who wish to follow a vegetarian diet.

Meal Plan

	MEAL	RECIPE	PAGE
DAY 1	BREAKFAST	Banana-Walnut Morning "Sundae"	76
	SNACK	Spicy Roasted Chickpeas	92
	LUNCH	Curried Carrot Soup with Basil	121
	DINNER	Quinoa "Tabbouleh"	142
DAY 2	BREAKFAST	Double-Boiler Scrambled Eggs	83
	SNACK	Crunchy Kale Chips	94
	LUNCH	Arugula and White Bean Salad	115
	DINNER	Ricotta-Stuffed Spaghetti Squash	134
DAY 3	BREAKFAST	Breakfast Grains with Hazelnuts	77
	SNACK	Lemon-Marinated Olives	98
	LUNCH	Quick Curried Lentil Stew	122
	DINNER	Spinach and White Bean Stew	148
DAY 4	BREAKFAST	Crustless Spring Quiche	86
	SNACK	Savory Couch Nuts	95
	LUNCH	Green Tea Smoothie	72
	DINNER	Ratatouille	144
DAY 5	BREAKFAST	Grain-Free Granola	79
	SNACK	No-Mayo Deviled Eggs	99
	LUNCH	Ratatouille-Stuffed Peppers	146
	DINNER	Grilled Portobello Mushrooms with Whipped Parsnips	128

MEAL	RECIPE	PAGE
DAY 6		
BREAKFAST	Mexican Eggs	87
SNACK	Strawberry-Almond Smoothie	73
LUNCH	Lemon and Arugula Pasta	130
DINNER	Asian Slaw with Thai Tofu	139
DAY 7		
BREAKFAST	Poached Eggs with Tomato, Basil, and Avocado	88
SNACK	Scallion Tofu Dip	102
LUNCH	Lemon-Lime Detox Smoothie	74
DINNER	Sesame-Ginger Soba Noodles	141
DAY 8		
BREAKFAST	Nutty Almond Butter–Banana Bites	75
SNACK	Roasted Edamame with Cracked Pepper	101
LUNCH	Sweet Pea Soup	119
DINNER	Lentil–Brown Rice Casserole	136
DAY 9		
BREAKFAST	Chocolate-Blackberry Frappé	70
SNACK	Savory Green Smoothie	71
LUNCH	Balsamic Quinoa-Spinach Salad	110
DINNER	Spiced Chickpeas with Grilled Tofu	137
DAY 10		
BREAKFAST	Grain-Free Granola	79
SNACK	Crunchy Kale Chips	94
LUNCH	Curried Carrot Soup with Basil	121
DINNER	Spinach and Feta Summer Squash "Pasta"	132

Shopping List

Fresh Produce and Herbs: Days 1–5

Arugula, 1 (6-ounce) bag
Avocado (1)
Banana, green-tipped (1)
Basil, fresh (1 small bunch)
Bell peppers, assorted colors (7)
Carrots (2)
Celery (1 stalk)
Cilantro, fresh (1 bunch)
Cucumber, English (1)
Eggplant (1)
Garlic (3 bulbs)
Ginger root (1 knob)
Kale (3 bunches)
Lemons (8)
Limes (2)
Mushrooms, portobello (4)
Onions, yellow (6)
Parsley, fresh (2 bunches)
Parsnips (4)
Scallions (1 bunch)
Spinach, baby, 1 (5-ounce) bag
Squash, spaghetti (1)
Squash, yellow (1)
Tomatoes (16)

Fresh Produce and Herbs: Days 6–10

Avocado (1)
Bananas, green-tipped (3)
Basil (1 bunch)
Bell peppers, red (1)

Cabbage, napa (1 head)
Cilantro (1 bunch)
Mushrooms, sliced, 1 (8-ounce) package
Oregano (1 bunch)
Pepper, jalapeño (1)
Scallions (1 bunch)
Spinach, baby, 1 (8-ounce) bag
Tomatoes (10)
Squash, yellow or zucchini (2)

Dairy and Eggs

Cheese, Cheddar (4 ounces)
Cheese, feta, crumbled, 1 (8-ounce) container
Cheese, mozzarella (2 ounces)
Cheese, Parmesan, grated (4 ounces)
Cheese, ricotta, 1 (12-ounce) container
Cream, heavy (½ pint)
Eggs (2 dozen)
Yogurt, Greek, plain, 1 (6-ounce) container

Frozen Foods

Blackberries (8 ounces)
Broccoli (10 ounces)
Carrots, chopped (16 ounces)
Edamame, shelled (16 ounces)
Peas, green (16 ounces)
Spinach (20 ounces)
Strawberries (8 ounces)

Pantry Items

Herbs and Spices
Bay leaf
Black pepper
Cayenne pepper
Cinnamon, ground
Cumin, ground
Curry powder
Ginger, ground
Mustard powder
Nutmeg, ground
Paprika
Red pepper flakes
Salt, coarse
Tarragon, dried

Oils and Vinegars
Oil, coconut
Oil, extra-virgin olive
Oil, sesame
Vinegar, balsamic
Vinegar, red wine
Vinegar, rice
Vinegar, white distilled

Nuts, Seeds, and Nut Butters
Almonds
Almond butter
Cashews
Coconut, unsweetened shredded
Flaxseed, ground
Hazelnuts
Pecans
Pistachios, shelled

Pumpkin seeds
Sesame seeds
Walnuts

Flours and Grains
Pasta, gluten-free
Rice, brown
Noodles, soba
Quinoa

Canned Goods
Chickpeas, 3 (15-ounce) cans
Cannellini beans,
    2 (15-ounce) cans
Coconut milk, 3 (15-ounce) cans
Lentils, 2 (15-ounce) cans

Other
Broth, vegetable,
    3 (32-ounce) cartons
Chia seeds
Cocoa powder
Milk, almond
Milk, coconut, unsweetened,
    1 (32-ounce) carton
Olives, green
Tamari, wheat-free
    (or coconut aminos)
Tea, green
Tofu, silken (4 ounces)
Tofu, extra-firm (16 ounces)
Vanilla extract
Worcestershire sauce,
    vegetarian

● YELLOW PLAN

When following the Yellow meal plan, you will consume meat, fish, and eggs; vegetables; nuts and seeds; and limited amounts of gluten-free grains and legumes and full-fat dairy.

Meal Plan

	MEAL	RECIPE	PAGE
DAY 1	BREAKFAST	Cheesy Bacon Breakfast Casserole	81
	SNACK	Spicy Roasted Chickpeas	92
	LUNCH	Sweet Pea Soup	119
	DINNER	Baked White Fish Fillets	158
DAY 2	BREAKFAST	Banana-Walnut Morning "Sundae"	76
	SNACK	Crunchy Kale Chips	94
	LUNCH	Chicken Salad with Walnuts	109
	DINNER	Creamy Spinach and Bacon Pie	177
DAY 3	BREAKFAST	Double-Boiler Scrambled Eggs	83
	SNACK	Homemade Hummus	97
	LUNCH	Guacamole Salad with Chicken	114
	DINNER	Shrimp Scampi	156
DAY 4	BREAKFAST	Egg and Prosciutto–Stuffed Mushroom Caps	84
	SNACK	Bacon-Wrapped Chicken Bites	96
	LUNCH	Quick Curried Lentil Stew	122
	DINNER	Hobo Packets	176
DAY 5	BREAKFAST	Breakfast Grains with Hazelnuts	77
	SNACK	Savory Couch Nuts	95
	LUNCH	Steak Salad with Goat Cheese	112
	DINNER	Ground Beef Casserole with Cheese Crust	183

MEAL	RECIPE	PAGE
BREAKFAST	Crustless Spring Quiche	86
SNACK	Lemon-Marinated Olives	98
LUNCH	Bacon and Broccoli Salad	108
DINNER	Meatballs, Your Way	182
BREAKFAST	Grain-Free Granola	79
SNACK	No-Mayo Deviled Eggs	99
LUNCH	Asian Slaw with Thai Tofu	139
DINNER	Curry-Ginger Pork Chops	178
BREAKFAST	Mexican Eggs	87
SNACK	Cucumber and Tuna Salad Bites	100
LUNCH	Lemon and Arugula Pasta	130
DINNER	Chile-Lime Grilled Salmon	160
BREAKFAST	Poached Eggs with Tomato, Basil, and Avocado	88
SNACK	Roasted Edamame with Cracked Pepper	101
LUNCH	Balsamic Quinoa-Spinach Salad	110
DINNER	Argentinean-Style Beef	181
BREAKFAST	Nutty Almond Butter–Banana Bites	75
SNACK	Scallion Tofu Dip	102
LUNCH	Bacon and Broccoli Salad	108
DINNER	Lemon-Thyme Roasted Chicken	174

Days (left vertical labels): DAY 6, DAY 7, DAY 8, DAY 9, DAY 10

Shopping List

Fresh Produce and Herbs: Days 1–5

Avocados (2)
Banana, green-tipped (1)
Basil (1 small bunch)
Carrot (1)
Celery (3 stalks)
Cilantro (1 small bunch)
Cucumber (1)
Dill (1 small bunch)
Garlic (1 bulb)
Ginger root (1 knob)
Kale (1 bunch)
Lemons (12)
Lettuce, romaine (2 heads)
Limes (3)
Mushrooms, portobello (2)
Onions, green (1 bunch)
Onion, red (1)
Onions, yellow (4)
Parsley (1 small bunch)
Salad greens (1½ pounds)
Spinach, baby (1 pound)
Tomato (1 large)

Fresh Produce and Herbs: Days 6–10

Arugula (1½ pounds)
Avocado (1)
Banana, green-tipped (1)
Bell pepper, green (1)
Bell pepper, red (1)
Broccoli (4 cups)
Cabbage, napa (1 head)
Cucumber, English (1 large)
Pepper, jalapeño (1)
Onions, green (3 bunches)

Spinach, baby (1½ pounds)
Thyme (4 sprigs)
Tomatoes (4 large)

Dairy and Eggs

Cheese, Cheddar (32 ounces)
Cheese, goat (2 ounces)
Cheese, Gruyère (6 ounces)
Cheese, Parmesan (6 ounces)
Cheese, Pecorino Romano
    (12 ounces)
Cream, heavy (1 pint)
Eggs (3 dozen)
Milk, whole (1 pint)
Sour cream (5 ounces)
Yogurt, Greek, plain (8 ounces)

Meat

Bacon (1 pound)
Beef, flank steak (1 pound)
Beef, ground (20 ounces)
Beef, sirloin (4 ounces)
Chicken breasts, boneless
    skinless (5)
Chicken, whole, 1 (5 to 6 pounds)
Fish, white, 2 (6-ounce) fillets
Pork chops, boneless, 2
    (6-ounce) chops
Prosciutto (2 ounces)
Salmon, 2 (6-ounce) fillets
Shrimp (12 ounces)

Frozen Foods

Broccoli (8 ounces)
Edamame, shelled (8 ounces)
Mixed vegetables (16 ounces)
Peas, green (1½ pounds)
Spinach (10 ounces)

Pantry Items

Herbs and Spices
Bay leaf
Black pepper
Cayenne pepper
Chili powder
Cinnamon, ground
Cumin, ground
Curry powder
Ginger, ground
Mustard powder
Nutmeg, ground
Paprika
Red pepper flakes
Salt
Tarragon, dried

Oils and Vinegars
Oil, coconut
Oil, extra-virgin olive
Oil, sesame
Vinegar, balsamic
Vinegar, red wine
Vinegar, rice
Vinegar, white

Nuts, Seeds, and Nut Butters
Almond butter
Almond flour
Almonds, raw
Coconut, unsweetened shredded
Flaxseed, ground
Hazelnuts, raw
Pecans, raw

Pistachios, shelled
Pumpkin seeds
Sesame seeds
Sunflower seeds, shelled
Tahini
Walnuts, raw

Flours and Grains
Pasta, gluten-free (4 ounces)
Quinoa (1 cup)

Canned Goods
Broth, chicken or vegetable
  (40 ounces)
Chickpeas, 4 (15-ounce) cans
Coconut milk, 3 (15-ounce) cans
Hearts of palm, 1 (15-ounce) can
Olives, green (1 pound)
Red peppers, roasted,
  1 (12-ounce) jar
Tuna, water packed,
  1 (6-ounce) can

Other
Anchovy fillets
Coconut aminos
Lentils (15 ounces)
Mustard, Dijon
Tofu, extra-firm (8 ounces)
Tofu, silken (4 ounces)
Tortilla chips, gluten-free, baked
Vanilla extract
Worcestershire sauce, vegetarian

GREEN PLAN

When following the Green meal plan, you will consume meat, fish, and eggs; vegetables; nuts and seeds; and limited amounts of full-fat dairy. This meal plan excludes all grains and legumes, even those that are gluten-free. The Green plan is recommended for individuals suffering from gluten sensitivities and those who have celiac disease.

Meal Plan

	MEAL	RECIPE	PAGE
DAY 1	BREAKFAST	Cheesy Bacon Breakfast Casserole	84
	SNACK	Lemon-Lime Detox Smoothie	74
	LUNCH	Pumpkin-Sage Soup	120
	DINNER	Baked White Fish Fillets	158
DAY 2	BREAKFAST	Banana-Walnut Morning "Sundae"	76
	SNACK	Crunchy Kale Chips	94
	LUNCH	Chicken Salad with Walnuts	109
	DINNER	Creamy Spinach and Bacon Pie	177
DAY 3	BREAKFAST	Double-Boiler Scrambled Eggs	83
	SNACK	Cucumber and Tuna Salad Bites	100
	LUNCH	Guacamole Salad with Chicken	114
	DINNER	Shrimp Scampi	156
DAY 4	BREAKFAST	Egg and Prosciutto–Stuffed Mushroom Caps	84
	SNACK	Bacon-Wrapped Chicken Bites	96
	LUNCH	Steak Salad with Goat Cheese	112
	DINNER	Hobo Packets	176
DAY 5	BREAKFAST	Savory Green Smoothie	71
	SNACK	Savory Couch Nuts	95
	LUNCH	Bacon and Broccoli Salad	108
	DINNER	Ground Beef Casserole with Cheese Crust	183

MEAL	RECIPE	PAGE
BREAKFAST	Crustless Spring Quiche	86
SNACK	Lemon-Marinated Olives	98
LUNCH	Savory Green Smoothie	71
DINNER	Meatballs, Your Way	182
BREAKFAST	Grain-Free Granola	79
SNACK	No-Mayo Deviled Eggs	99
LUNCH	Pumpkin-Sage Soup	120
DINNER	Curry-Ginger Pork Chops	178
BREAKFAST	Mexican Eggs	87
SNACK	Cucumber and Tuna Salad Bites	100
LUNCH	Chicken Salad with Walnuts	109
DINNER	Chile-Lime Grilled Salmon	160
BREAKFAST	Poached Eggs with Tomato, Basil, and Avocado	88
SNACK	Crunchy Kale Chips	94
LUNCH	Curried Carrot Soup with Basil	121
DINNER	Argentinean-Style Beef	181
BREAKFAST	Nutty Almond Butter–Banana Bites	75
SNACK	Bacon-Wrapped Chicken Bites	96
LUNCH	Bacon and Broccoli Salad	108
DINNER	Lemon-Thyme Roasted Chicken	174

(Rows grouped by DAY 6, DAY 7, DAY 8, DAY 9, DAY 10 respectively.)

Shopping List

Fresh Produce and Herbs: Days 1–5

Avocados (2)
Bananas, green-tipped (3)
Basil (1 small bunch)
Celery (6 stalks)
Cilantro (1 small bunch)
Cucumber (1)
Cucumber, English (1 large)
Dill (1 small bunch)
Garlic (1 bulb)
Ginger root (1 large knob)
Kale (2 bunches)
Lemons (10)
Lettuce, romaine (2 heads)
Limes (3)
Mushrooms, portobello (2)
Onions, green (1 bunch)
Onion, red (1)
Onions, yellow (3)
Parsley (1 small bunch)
Sage (1 small bunch)
Salad greens, mixed (3 cups)
Spinach, baby (1 pound)
Tomatoes (3 large)

Fresh Produce and Herbs: Days 6–10

Avocados (2)
Bananas, green-tipped (2)
Basil (1 bunch)
Bell pepper, green (1)
Broccoli (1 pound)
Celery (6 stalks)
Cilantro (1 bunch)
Cucumber, English (1)
Dill (1 bunch)
Garlic (1 bulb)
Kale (2 bunches)

Oregano (1 small bunch)
Parsley (1 bunch)
Pepper, jalapeño (1)
Thyme (1 small bunch)
Tomatoes (2 large, 1 small)

Dairy and Eggs

Cheese, Cheddar (16 ounces)
Cheese, goat (2 ounces)
Cheese, Gruyère (12 ounces)
Cheese, Parmesan (8 ounces)
Cheese, Pecorino Romano
    (12 ounces)
Cream, heavy (1 pint)
Eggs (4 dozen)
Milk, whole (12 ounces)
Sour cream (5 ounces)
Yogurt, Greek, plain (8 ounces)

Meat

Bacon, thick cut (2 pounds)
Beef, flank steak (20 ounces)
Beef, lean ground (20 ounces)
Chicken breast, boneless and
    skinless (3 pounds)
Chicken, whole, 1 (5 to 6 pounds)
Fish, haddock or cod, 2 (6-ounce)
    white fillets
Pork chops, boneless,
    2 (6-ounce) chops
Prosciutto (2 ounces)
Salmon, 2 (6-ounce) fillets
Shrimp (12 ounces)

Frozen Foods

Broccoli (8 ounces)
Carrots (16 ounces)
Mixed vegetables (16 ounces)
Peas, green (8 ounces)

Pantry Items

Herbs and Spices

Black pepper
Cayenne pepper
Chili powder
Cinnamon, ground
Cumin, ground
Curry powder
Mustard powder
Nutmeg, ground
Paprika
Red pepper flakes
Salt
Tarragon, dried

Oils and Vinegars

Oil, coconut
Oil, extra-virgin olive
Vinegar, red wine
Vinegar, white

Nuts, Seeds, and Nut Butters

Almond butter
Almonds, raw
Chia seeds
Coconut, unsweetened shredded
Flaxseed, ground
Hazelnuts, raw
Pecans, raw
Pistachios, shelled
Pumpkin seeds
Sunflower seeds, raw
Walnuts, raw

Canned Goods

Anchovy fillets (4)
Broth, vegetable or chicken
    (48 ounces)
Coconut milk, 3 (15-ounce) cans
Hearts of palm, 1 (15-ounce) can
Olives, green (16 ounces)
Pumpkin puree, 1 (15-ounce) can
Tuna, water-packed,
    2 (6-ounce) cans

Other

Cooking spray
Roasted red peppers,
    1 (12-ounce) jar
Tortilla chips, gluten-free, baked
Vanilla extract
Worcestershire sauce

● BLUE PLAN

When following the Blue meal plan, you will consume meat, fish, and eggs; vegetables; and nuts and seeds. The Blue plan excludes all dairy and all grains and legumes, including those that are gluten-free. This plan has the most restrictions of the four and is intended for those who wish to follow a high-protein, low-carb, or Paleo-style diet.

Meal Plan

	MEAL	RECIPE	PAGE
DAY 1	BREAKFAST	Poached Eggs with Tomato, Basil, and Avocado	88
	SNACK	Lemon-Lime Detox Smoothie	74
	LUNCH	Curried Carrot Soup with Basil	121
	DINNER	Ratatouille (omit cheese)	144
DAY 2	BREAKFAST	Banana-Walnut Morning "Sundae"	76
	SNACK	Crunchy Kale Chips	94
	LUNCH	Bacon-Wrapped Chicken Bites	96
	DINNER	Chile-Lime Grilled Salmon	160
DAY 3	BREAKFAST	Grain-Free Granola	79
	SNACK	Cucumber and Tuna Salad Bites	100
	LUNCH	Lemon-Lime Detox Smoothie	74
	DINNER	Argentinean-Style Beef	181
DAY 4	BREAKFAST	Egg and Prosciutto–Stuffed Mushroom Caps	84
	SNACK	Bacon-Wrapped Chicken Bites	96
	LUNCH	Cucumber and Tuna Salad Bites (left over from day 3)	100
	DINNER	Hobo Packets	176
DAY 5	BREAKFAST	Savory Green Smoothie	71
	SNACK	Savory Couch Nuts	95
	LUNCH	Curried Carrot Soup with Basil	121
	DINNER	Lemon-Thyme Roasted Chicken	174

	MEAL	RECIPE	PAGE
DAY 6	BREAKFAST	Nutty Almond Butter–Banana Bites	75
	SNACK	Lemon-Marinated Olives	98
	LUNCH	Strawberry-Almond Smoothie	73
	DINNER	Meatballs, Your Way (omit cheese)	182
DAY 7	BREAKFAST	Grain-Free Granola	79
	SNACK	No-Mayo Deviled Eggs	99
	LUNCH	Pumpkin-Sage Soup	120
	DINNER	Curry-Ginger Pork Chops	178
DAY 8	BREAKFAST	Banana-Walnut Morning "Sundae"	76
	SNACK	Cucumber and Tuna Salad Bites	100
	LUNCH	Bacon-Wrapped Chicken Bites	96
	DINNER	Chicken Fajita Lettuce Cups	175
DAY 9	BREAKFAST	Poached Eggs with Tomato, Basil, and Avocado	88
	SNACK	Crunchy Kale Chips	94
	LUNCH	Cucumber and Tuna Salad Bites (left over from day 8)	100
	DINNER	Herb-Marinated Cod	162
DAY 10	BREAKFAST	Nutty Almond Butter–Banana Bites	75
	SNACK	Bacon-Wrapped Chicken Bites	96
	LUNCH	Green Tea Smoothie	72
	DINNER	Grilled Garlic-Rosemary Pork Tenderloin with Steamed Broccoli	179

Shopping List

Fresh Produce and Herbs:
Days 1–5
Avocado (1)
Bananas, green-tipped (4)
Basil (2 bunches)
Cucumber, English (1 large)
Eggplant (1 large)
Garlic (2 bulbs)
Ginger root (1 large knob)
Kale (2 bunches)
Lemons (11)
Limes (5)
Mushrooms, portobello (2)
Onion, red (1)
Onions, yellow (4)
Parsley (1 small bunch)
Sage (1 bunch)
Spinach, baby (1½ pounds)
Squash, yellow (1 large)
Tomatoes (2 pounds)

Fresh Produce and Herbs:
Days 6–10
Avocado (1)
Bananas, green-tipped (3)
Basil (1 large bunch)
Bell peppers, any color (2)
Broccoli (1½ pounds)
Cucumber, English (1 large)
Kale (1 bunch)
Lettuce (1 head)

Oregano (1 bunch)
Rosemary (1 bunch)
Sage (1 bunch)
Spinach, baby (8 ounces)
Tarragon (1 bunch)
Thyme (1 small bunch)
Tomato (1 large)

Dairy and Eggs
Almond milk, unsweetened
    (1 pint)
Eggs (2 dozen)

Meat
Bacon (1 pound)
Beef, flank steak (1 pound)
Beef, lean ground (12 ounces)
Chicken, boneless and skinless
    (3½ pounds)
Chicken, whole, 1 (5 to 6 pounds)
Cod (12 ounces)
Pork chops, boneless,
    2 (6-ounce) chops
Pork tenderloin (1 pound)
Prosciutto (2 ounces)
Salmon, 2 (6-ounce) fillets

Frozen Foods
Carrots (32 ounces)
Mixed vegetables (16 ounces)
Strawberries (8 ounces)

Pantry Items

Herbs and Spices
Black pepper
Cayenne pepper
Chili powder
Cinnamon, ground
Cumin, ground
Curry powder
Mustard powder
Nutmeg, ground
Paprika
Red pepper flakes
Salt
Tarragon, dried

Oils and Vinegars
Oil, coconut
Oil, extra-virgin olive
Vinegar, red wine
Vinegar, rice
Vinegar, white

Nuts, Seeds, and Nut Butters
Almonds, raw
Almond butter
Almond flour
Cashews
Chia seeds
Coconut, unsweetened shredded
Flaxseed
Hazelnuts
Pecans, raw
Pistachios, shelled
Pumpkin seeds
Sunflower seeds, raw and hulled
Walnuts, raw

Canned Goods
Broth, vegetable or chicken
   (10 cups)
Coconut milk, 6 (15-ounce) cans
Olives, green (16 ounces)
Pumpkin puree, 2 (15-ounce) cans
Tuna, 2 (6-ounce) cans

Other
Coconut aminos
Tea, green
Vanilla extract
Worcestershire sauce

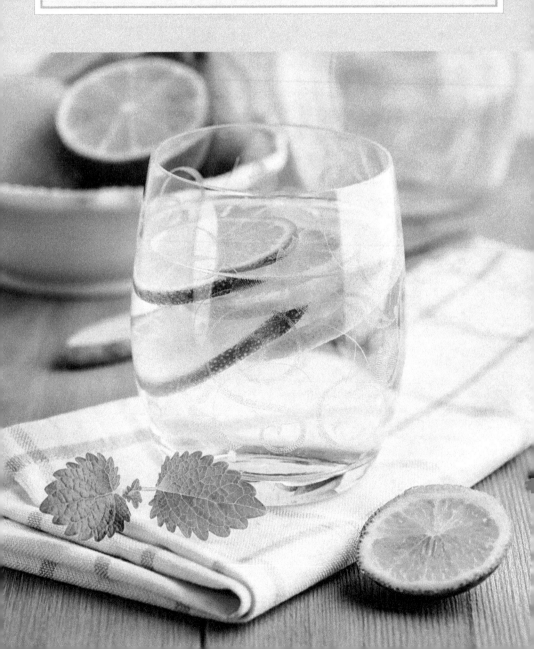

FOUR

PREPARING FOR
YOUR DETOX

While a 10-day commitment might not seem all that daunting, a detox of any kind or time span requires a certain amount of preparation. In order to be successful, you have to properly prepare your home and your body so you can focus on the detox and be free from distractions. If you spend the time to ready yourself for change, you will receive optimum results from the detox.

Preparing Your Kitchen

Since you are detoxing your body of sugar, you need to do the same for your kitchen. By removing all sugar-laden foods and products, you can eliminate temptations that can interfere with your meal plan.

What to Avoid

Before you start your detox, take an inventory of your kitchen. Read the labels of everything you find, and get rid of anything that contains added sugars. If you're doing a detox that does not allow grains, rice, beans, or legumes, you'll also want to toss or stash those items out of sight to reduce temptation. Here are some common pantry items that are especially high in added sugar and should be evicted from your kitchen while you are on the 10-day detox:

- Sweetened drinks like juice, soda, and sports beverages
- Alcohol
- Sugary breakfast cereals (think Froot Loops and Frosted Flakes)
- Every kind of artificial sweetener
- Anything containing gluten, which includes all wheat-based products such as bread, pasta, bagels, crackers, and muffins.
- Caffeine (coffee and caffeinated tea)
- Honey, molasses, and maple sugar
- Anything containing hydrogenated oils or refined vegetable oils

Now open your refrigerator. Some foods that you see in there will be used sparingly, if at all, on your detox. Remove these foods from the fridge or push them to the back of the shelves, out of sight:

- Milk
- Yogurt
- Butter
- Cheese
- Store-bought condiments, such as ketchup, mayonnaise, and relish
- Store-bought salad dressings

Kitchen Prep Checklist:
"No" Foods for the Next 10 Days

AVOID ON ALL DETOXES

- Alcohol (wine, beer, spirits)
- Bagels
- Bread
- Canned fruit
- Canned soup
- Cereal
- Chocolate
- Coffee
- Crackers
- Cream sauce
- Dried fruit
- Fruit juice
- Granola
- Honey
- Instant oatmeal
- Jams and jellies
- Maple syrup

- Nonfat and low-fat dairy products
- Pasta made with refined flour
- Pasta sauce
- Popcorn
- Potato chips
- Processed cheese
- Refined flour
- Rice cakes
- Soda
- Soy sauce
- Store-bought condiments (including ketchup, mayonnaise, relish, and salad dressings)
- Tea (other than herbal caffeine-free)
- White potatoes
- White rice

AVOID ON THE ORANGE PLAN

- Fish and seafood
- Meat

AVOID ON THE GREEN PLAN

- Beans
- Black-eyed peas
- Brown rice
- Corn (including corn grits and popcorn)
- Flours made from grains
- Green peas
- Lentils
- Oats
- Quinoa
- Soy products
- Wild rice

AVOID ON THE BLUE PLAN

- Beans: black, garbanzo, kidney, pinto
- Black-eyed peas
- Brown rice
- Corn (including corn grits and popcorn)
- Dairy
- Flours made from grains
- Green peas
- Lentils
- Oats
- Quinoa
- Soy products
- Wheat
- Wild rice

Once you've rid your kitchen of high-sugar foods and ingredients, you may notice that there's not much left. Put the high-sugar food items in a box and donate any unopened containers to your local food bank. Or, if your family won't be observing the diet, try to organize a section of your pantry that's free of these items, and clear out a "sugar-free" shelf in your fridge, so you won't be tempted to cheat during the detox. After the 10 days are up, you can reintroduce some of these items to your kitchen on a gradual and smaller scale—that is, if you still have an appetite for them at all.

During the 10-Day Sugar Detox, you will be introducing better foods and ingredients to your diet that are proven to help break sugar addiction and detoxify the body. As you follow the meal plans and use the shopping lists included in this chapter, your fridge and pantry will reflect a much healthier lifestyle.

A Word About Equipment

Removing sugar from your diet requires no special equipment. Most likely, you already have the basic tools you need for a successful detox:

- Food processor
- Mixing bowls
- Pots and pans with thick, heat-conducting bases so that food cooks evenly
- Sharp chef's knife
- Sharp paring knife

A refurbished brand-name food processor can be bought for as little as $40 and will work like new.

An electric coffee grinder is about $20 and is wonderful for grinding spices and seeds. Just make sure you wash it well between uses if you also plan on grinding coffee beans.

In several recipes, an electric handheld mixer is used; this tool is available online for less than $15.

Preparing Your Body

Going "cold turkey" has its advantages and can be effective for some people, but more often than not, this approach ends up failing. Remember, your body has been consuming high amounts of sugar for a long time, and from various sources. It's used to receiving it every day and relies on it for an energy source. If you pull the plug on sugar too abruptly, you will probably face severe withdrawal symptoms and end up abandoning your detox before you've even begun.

To avoid serious withdrawal symptoms, begin to slowly wean yourself off of sugar about three days before your detox begins. Focus on consuming half your usual amounts of caffeine, alcohol, and sugar. For example, if you always drink two cups of coffee in the morning, cut that down to just one. If your regular lunch includes a PB&J, use only half the usual amount of jam. Don't worry too much about the sugar you may eat here and there; instead, focus on identifying the sugar sources in your daily life. These probably will be where most of your sugar consumption comes from, and reducing your intake by 50 percent will help you make great strides toward breaking your habit.

Also, begin to increase your intake of noncaffeinated fluids. Begin each morning with 16 ounces of hot water with lemon, and drink one cup of caffeine-free herbal tea before bed. During the day, drink at least eight glasses of water. Here are a few more ways to prepare your body for a sugar detox:

- Schedule the beginning of your detox over a weekend. You might want to clear your calendar of social engagements for the 10 days. It's not because you need to sequester yourself to succeed; limiting situations that will tempt you to cheat simply makes it easier on you. This way you can ease into the detox process before venturing back into your everyday life.

- Avoid any heavy physical activity or arduous tasks during the detox's initial days. You want to keep your energy levels as high as possible, so refrain from doing any housework or chores. Keep everything simple and stress-free.

- Before beginning the detox, buy all of your pantry items and as many of the grocery items as makes sense. Keep in mind that you might need to make two shopping trips, as fresh fruits and vegetables are unlikely to last all 10 days.

- Start a journal to record your feelings and experiences. Journaling can be a strong support tool to help you navigate through rough spots—and also to celebrate your victories, which can be easy to forget during more challenging moments.

- If you're receptive to it, try to meditate or sit quietly for at least 10 minutes a day leading up to your detox, and continue this practice every day during the 10-day detox period. It's important to support your mind as you work to detox your body.

- Clean your home of all clutter, messes, and distractions before you begin the detox. A clean, comfortable space will help reduce stress and promote a relaxing atmosphere.

- Make sure you have a stockpile of brain candy on hand. When your mind wanders to thoughts of sugar during the detox, turn on some music, start a new book, begin a crossword puzzle, or pop in your favorite movie. These distracters will divert your attention and stave off temptation.

What Your Body Can Expect When Quitting Sugar

Each person will react differently to a sugar detox. Some may not notice any major changes, while others will experience various forms of withdrawal. Where you will fall on the spectrum depends on the level of your sugar addiction, your current health, and whether you are a big consumer of caffeine.

DAYS 1 THROUGH 3: During the early stages of the detox, the most common symptoms include cravings for sweets that may become intense, especially if you are used to certain high-sugar foods or beverages at specific times of the day—for instance, that 2 p.m. vending-machine snack or late-afternoon can of Coke. This may trigger an occasional headache and a feeling of nausea or diarrhea as your body copes with the sudden lack of sugar intake.

DAYS 4 THROUGH 6: At the halfway point, you may encounter old symptoms, new ones, or various combinations. Your cravings may continue as before, but with less frequency and intensity. You also may experience a little fatigue and mental fogginess.

DAYS 7 THROUGH 9: By now your cravings have likely reduced and you are probably feeling pretty good about yourself (or at least you should be). A little fatigue may still be lingering, but not to worry: By the time you complete the detox, the elation you'll feel will perk you up.

DAY 10: On your last day, you should be almost free of negative symptoms (if you had any at all). You might feel a bit nervous about what to eat next and how to start planning your own meals. Keep in mind that the recipe section of this book contains enough recipes to carry you well past 10 days. Flip through and revisit your favorites or try new ones.

Psychological Effects of Addiction Withdrawal

If you are highly dependent on refined sugar or artificial sweeteners, you may experience withdrawal symptoms often found in drug abusers, such as fatigue, anxiety and irritability, depression and detachment, rapid heart rate, and poor sleep. This may sound strange, but as mentioned briefly in chapter 2, research has found that drug and sugar addictions share the same psychological effects.

According to a study conducted at Princeton University, rats that ate large amounts of sugar when hungry, a phenomenon described as sugar bingeing, underwent neurochemical changes in the brain that mimic those produced by highly addictive substances such as cocaine, morphine, and nicotine. The experts found that dopamine, a feel-good brain chemical, was released when the rats drank a sugar solution. Dopamine can trigger motivation, which can lead to repetition and eventually addiction, according to the researchers.

When the rats' sugar solution was suddenly reintroduced after a period of restriction, they dove into binge eating, consuming as much sugar as they could at one time and demonstrating neurological signs of substance abuse. When their sugar supply was taken away, the rats also exhibited classic signs of withdrawal—anxiety, nervousness, and social isolation—which further supported the researchers' theory that sugar is in fact an addictive substance.

Don't be alarmed if you begin to experience strong cravings for sugar or withdrawal symptoms during your 10-day detox. Keep in mind that these reactions are normal and will eventually subside as your body begins to adjust to restricted amounts of sugar. There is no set order in which the symptoms may appear, if they appear at all, so it's best to just be mindful that they could occur and prepare to manage them when they arise.

One way to cope with persistent cravings is by increasing your water intake. Often when people crave sugary foods it is actually because their bodies are thirsty, and they have trouble identifying the difference. So when you feel a sugar urge, drink a glass of water. In a 2010 study, the American Chemical Society found that just 16 ounces of water can suppress the appetite when taken before meals and reduce the risk of overeating.

Another way to combat cravings is with exercise. When your mind wanders to thoughts of sugary foods, respond with some kind of physical activity, which can also help regulate the mood changes associated with common withdrawal symptoms. While conducting a study on the relationship between exercise and nicotine addiction, which was published in the scientific journal *Psychopharmacology*, researchers found that short bouts (10 minutes) of moderate to intense exercise can reduce withdrawal symptoms and cravings. Further studies have concluded that the chemical galanin, found in the brain during exercise, appears to lower certain stress-related cravings, and intense exercise can also trigger the brain's release of endorphins and endocannabinoids, which can result in a natural high and a sense of calm.

Daily Detox Tracker

For many people, sticking to a detox is the most difficult part. If you have evidence of your progress right in front of you, however, you may find that you are more motivated to keep going even on your most challenging days. Use this work sheet to track your progress so you can see how far you have truly come. Before you begin, photocopy the page ten times so you have one for each day of the detox.

DAY # _____

SLEEP

Time to bed _____

This morning I felt (circle all that apply):
○ energized   ○ rested   ○ groggy   ○ tired   ○ exhausted

EXERCISE LOG

Type of exercise _____

Length of exercise _____

MOOD ASSESSMENT

Today I feel (circle all that apply):   ○ calm   ○ irritable   ○ impatient
○ nervous   ○ depressed   ○ content   ○ happy

FOOD LOG

Breakfast _____

Lunch _____

Snacks _____

Dinner _____

Dessert _____

ADDITIONAL NOTES

_____

_____

_____

FIVE

AFTER THE DETOX

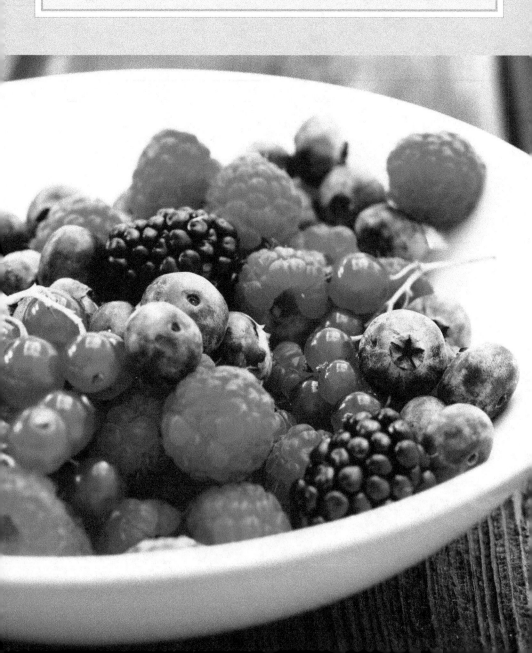

At the completion of the detox, you may already be experiencing the short-term benefits, including increased energy, clearer thinking, better sleep, and even weight loss. Most importantly, you'll have introduced new and healthier eating habits—habits that will have enabled you to break your sugar addiction and allowed your body a physical restart.

You have made a lot of progress in only 10 days, but what now? Where do you go from here?

First, let's take a look at some of your accomplishments over the last 10 days:

1. You realized you have the initiative to break your sugar habit. That is not easy to do, and making the commitment to change your health in order to live better should be commended.

2. You cut out all sources of sugar from your diet. You detoxified your kitchen to remove all foods that contain high amounts of sugar, including the hidden, sneaky kind.

3. You have introduced foods and ingredients to your diet that have helped your detoxification process, flushed out toxins, and jump-started your body's healing.

4. You have witnessed how you can live without a dependency on sugar and the positive effects it can have on your health and life.

When people follow a structured plan, they are more successful at reaching their goals. But eventually they have to go it alone and apply what they have learned and experienced to their daily lives. For some this can be difficult as they lose their momentum and focus and gradually slip back into their old habits. The 10-Day Sugar Detox has shown you how to break free of sugar; now it's up to you to continue these new habits as you move forward.

How to Stay Sugar-Free

During the detox, you probably discovered where your biggest sugar sources lie—from the seemingly innocent tablespoons of table sugar to your penchant for afternoon soft drinks. The key to staying sugar free after your detox is to continue focusing on those individual trouble spots to ensure that you don't slip back into bad habits. Here are some tips for keeping sugar at bay:

1. *Fight cravings with protein.* Your main obstacle now will be fighting off sugar cravings. Even if you think you have them under control, they will sneak up at unexpected times and test your will power. Don't let cravings control you. Instead, focus on preventing them from ever occurring. You can do this with protein, which can help balance blood sugar and insulin and thus reduce cravings. Try to incorporate a good amount of protein into every meal: Nuts, seeds, eggs, lean chicken, and grass-fed meat are some healthy options. Aim for a single serving size of 4 to 6 ounces, or about what can fit in the palm of your hand.

2. *Increase your intake of "good" carbs.* Up your intake of the good, complex carbohydrates—for instance, whole-grain products like brown rice, whole-grain pasta, beans, whole-wheat bread, whole oats, and buckwheat. But also include high amounts of nonstarchy vegetables, such as broccoli, cauliflower, asparagus, green beans, mushrooms, and zucchini. These are full of essential vitamins, minerals, and fiber and will help fill you up and provide energy without the need for quick-hit energy sources found in simple carbs.

3. *Don't drink your sugar.* No soda, sports drinks, sweetened teas, or mocha/latte beverages that are loaded with sugar. Instead, opt for a glass of water, maybe with a wedge of lemon or lime or a few slices of cucumber. Even adding a splash of fruit juice to water is absolutely fine—just make sure you've got a ratio of at least two-thirds water to one-third juice. Stick with your regular coffee and tea, but refrain from using more than a little natural sweetener (such as milk or honey), and no artificial sweeteners. If it's too bitter, try diluting it and see if that helps.

4. *Get some sleep.* If you had trouble sleeping in the past, you may have noticed a change in your slumber habits while on the 10-Day Sugar Detox. Many people who cut out sugar in their diets have an easier time falling asleep, and more

importantly, staying asleep. To keep your cravings under control, you need to continue a healthy sleep cycle. Everyone has different standards of what is adequate, but the ideal range is seven to eight hours per night. Get your proper sleep, and you can increase your production of appetite-suppressing hormones that can block out sugar cravings. Plus, according to a 2013 study from the University of California, Berkeley, sleep deprivation can cause an increase in desire for junk food and sweets.

Reintroducing Sugar into Your Diet

Once you have kicked the sugar habit, you may discover that you've lost your appetite for certain highly sweetened beverages or treats. However, if you find yourself missing other sources of sugar, like the spoonful of honey in your morning tea, you can reintroduce these indulgences in increments without compromising your now-detoxified body. Just increase your sugar intake little by very little, and monitor how you react and feel during this process.

For instance, during the detox you cut out all jams and jellies from your diet. Now you can add them back at a smaller dosage. Use only half a spoonful on your toast, and perhaps just on the weekend. Stir in only one teaspoon of sugar instead of your usual two for your morning cup of joe. You get the idea. The point is to be mindful about your sugar and realize how much you reintroduce into your routine. You'll find that you feel just as satisfied with half of your usual portions, and you won't experience those pesky cravings for more sweets throughout the day.

Dining Out

While you can control what goes into the foods you eat at home and take with you to work, it can be difficult to know what's in your food when you eat out at restaurants or other people's homes. Here are some suggestions for reducing your sugar intake when dining out:

1. *Make the choice.* Sometimes where to eat out is a group discussion. Take the lead. Find a place that you enjoy and that has a wide range of meals, including some low-sugar options.

2. *Don't arrive hungry.* This is popular advice for grocery shopping to prevent binge purchases, but it works in restaurants, too. If you arrive super hungry, you'll likely go for the sweet and bad carb selections, and probably overeat. Eat a snack beforehand. You won't ruin your appetite, and it will protect you from eyeing the sugary items on the menu.

3. *Drink your water.* Drink water before and during your meals to help curb your appetite and keep you from reaching for sugar- and carb-filled beverages like soda, beer, and cocktails.

4. *Embrace the salad course.* You can order some version of salad almost anywhere. There is nothing wrong with a rich salad full of vegetables as a main meal. Just remember to ask for sugar-free oil and vinegar (on the side) instead of the traditional dressings like ranch, Thousand Island, honey mustard, etc., which are all full of added sugar.

Sugar in Common Menu Items

The good news is that many eateries now offer nutritional breakdowns of their meals so you can gauge how much sugar they contain. As a general rule, any food or meal that contains more than 15 grams of sugar per serving is similar to a dessert, according to Marion Nestle, a nutrition professor at New York University. If there is no nutritional breakdown available, here are some tips on how to recognize sugary menu items in different types of restaurants:

ASIAN. Sugar is often hidden in sauces and dressings, especially anything with "sweet" in the title. Ask your server if any sweet sauces or dressings come with your meal, and if so, ask him or her to take it off (you won't need it for flavor) or serve it on the side.

DELI. The main culprits here are processed soups and any dressings or condiments. Lower your intake by opting for half servings and asking for condiments and sauces to be served on the side so you can add them yourself.

ITALIAN. Tomato sauces are often full of sugar. It's tough to avoid all sauces while eating Italian, but ask for a half portion of sauce, ask if they have no-sugar substitutes, or request that your sauce be served on the side. Sauces are often one of the last items added to entrées, so this shouldn't be difficult.

PIZZA. There is sugar in the dough, but as with Italian foods, the sauce is what you need to avoid. Request that they go light on the sauce, or better yet, skip it altogether and ask them to replace it with extra veggies.

Revisiting the Detox

One of the best things about this sugar detox is that you can revisit it whenever possible. Since it is set up for only a 10-day period, and you're already familiar with how it works, it will be much easier to adapt to it a second time.

There may be times when you find yourself slipping back into your sugar habits and need to break them again before they return to their full force. You might begin to feel the effects of your returning sugar addiction in the form of poor sleep or lack of energy, or you might begin to notice that your body has become more prone to colds and other illnesses.

But you don't have to wait until you feel something negative to rejuvenate your body with another 10-day detox. Use the sugar detox as part of your ongoing maintenance for your new healthy lifestyle. Try it again every two to three months as a general cleanse for your body. Or start a new detox whenever you feel the need for a physical and mental boost.

With four color-coded meal plans and 105 sugar-free recipes, this book includes everything you need to kick your sugar habit and make detoxing a part of your life. Going sugar-free has never been so sweet.

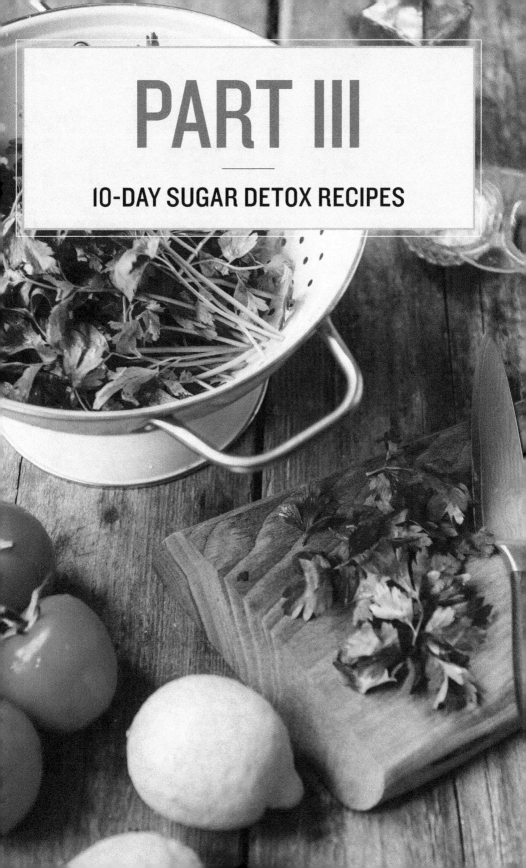

PART III

10-DAY SUGAR DETOX RECIPES

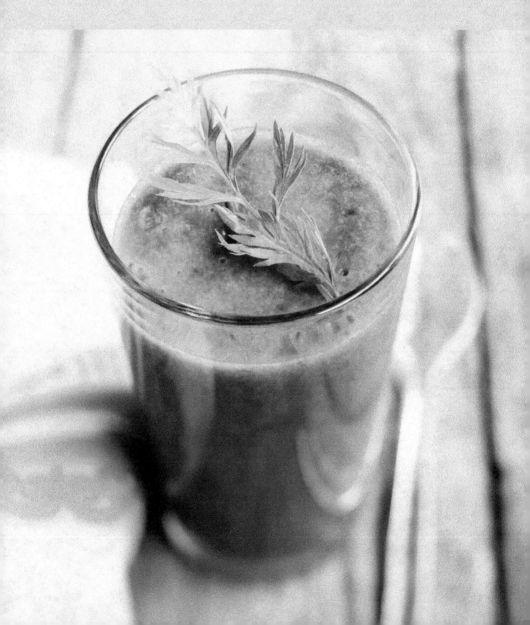

SIX

BREAKFAST

Chocolate-Blackberry Frappé 70

Savory Green Smoothie 71

Green Tea Smoothie 72

Strawberry-Almond Smoothie 73

Lemon-Lime Detox Smoothie 74

Nutty Almond Butter–Banana Bites 75

Banana-Walnut Morning "Sundae" 76

Breakfast Grains with Hazelnuts 77

Grain-Free Granola 79

Cheesy Bacon Breakfast Casserole 81

Double-Boiler Scrambled Eggs 83

Egg and Prosciutto–Stuffed Mushroom Caps 84

Crustless Spring Quiche 86

Mexican Eggs 87

Poached Eggs with Tomato, Basil, and Avocado 88

Chocolate-Blackberry Frappé

SERVES I PREP TIME: 5 MINUTES

MEAL PLAN ● ○ ○ ●

In this recipe, frozen blackberries do more than give your beverage a naturally sweet and refreshing flavor—they also add to the nutrient profile of the recipe. Blackberries contain anthocyanins, which have been shown to reduce inflammation and promote heart health. These berries are also a good source of vitamin C and phytoestrogens.

1 cup unsweetened coconut milk
½ cup frozen blackberries
2 tablespoons ground flaxseed
1 tablespoon unsweetened cocoa powder
2 or 3 ice cubes

1. In a blender, combine the coconut milk, blackberries, flaxseed, cocoa powder, and ice cubes.

2. Blend on high speed for 20 to 40 seconds until smooth and well combined.

3. Pour into a glass and serve immediately.

NUTRITION INFO Calories 162, Total Fat 10g, Carbohydrates 16g, Protein 5g, Cholesterol 0mg

Savory Green Smoothie

SERVES I   PREP TIME: 5 MINUTES
MEAL PLAN ● ○ ○ ●

Leafy greens like spinach and kale are jam-packed with nutrients while being very low in calories. These vegetables have high levels of dietary fiber, which is essential for healthy digestion—and they're also loaded with vitamin C and antioxidants, including lutein and zeaxanthin.

½ frozen green-tipped banana, sliced

1 small ripe tomato, chopped

½ cup fresh baby spinach leaves, packed

½ cup chopped kale leaves

½ ripe avocado, pitted and chopped

2 tablespoons chia seeds

1 tablespoon freshly squeezed lemon juice

2 or 3 ice cubes

1. In a blender, combine the banana, tomato, spinach, kale, avocado, chia seeds, lemon juice, and ice cubes.

2. Blend on high speed for 20 to 40 seconds until smooth and well combined.

3. Pour into a glass and serve immediately.

NUTRITION INFO Calories 355, Total Fat 25g, Carbohydrates 36g, Protein 8g, Cholesterol 0mg

TIP If you want to give your smoothie a thicker consistency without adding more ice, simply let the smoothie sit for a few minutes before you drink it. The chia seeds will absorb the liquid from the other ingredients and make the smoothie thicker.

Green Tea Smoothie

SERVES I   PREP TIME: 5 MINUTES
MEAL PLAN ● ● ● ●

Green tea is loaded with antioxidants that help protect your body against free-radical damage. It also contains a wide nutrient profile that has been shown to help improve brain function, speed fat loss, and reduce your risk for certain types of cancer.

> 2 cups brewed green tea, cooled to room temperature
> 1 cup fresh baby spinach leaves, packed
> ½ ripe avocado, pitted and chopped
> Pinch of salt
> 2 or 3 ice cubes

1. In a blender, combine the tea, spinach, avocado, salt, and ice cubes.

2. Blend on high speed for 20 to 40 seconds until smooth and well combined.

3. Pour into a glass and serve immediately.

NUTRITION INFO Calories 212, Total Fat 20g, Carbohydrates 10g, Protein 3g, Cholesterol 0mg

TIP To make your green tea for this recipe, simply steep a green tea bag in 2 cups of hot water for several minutes until brewed to the desired strength. Let the tea cool to room temperature before using it in your smoothie.

Strawberry Almond Smoothie

SERVES I   PREP TIME: 5 MINUTES
MEAL PLAN ● ○ ○ ○

Almonds have a light, versatile flavor that pairs well with the straw-berries in this recipe. In addition to their delicious flavor, almonds also contain high levels of vitamin E, copper, and manganese. In fact, a single ¼-cup serving of almonds contains about 40 percent of your daily value for vitamin E.

1 cup frozen strawberries
1 cup unsweetened almond milk
½ cup chopped almonds
2 tablespoons ground flaxseed
½ teaspoon ground cinnamon
2 or 3 ice cubes

1. In a blender, combine the strawberries, milk, almonds, flaxseed, cinnamon, and ice cubes.

2. Blend on high speed for 20 to 40 seconds until smooth and well combined.

3. Pour into a glass and serve immediately.

NUTRITION INFO Calories 432, Total Fat 31g, Carbohydrates 29g, Protein 14g, Cholesterol 0mg

Lemon-Lime Detox Smoothie

SERVES I   PREP TIME: 5 MINUTES
MEAL PLAN ● ○ ○ ○ ●

Lemon and lime have long been known for their beneficial detox qualities. Drinking lemon juice in water helps stimulate bile production, which is essential for detoxifying the liver. Lemon is also full of vitamin C, which helps speed healing and regeneration.

1 frozen green-tipped banana, sliced

1 cup water

1 cup chopped fresh kale leaves

Juice of ½ lime

Juice of ½ lemon

1 teaspoon freshly grated lemon zest

2 or 3 ice cubes (optional)

1. In a blender, combine the banana, water, kale, lime and lemon juices, lemon zest, and ice cubes (if using).

2. Blend on high speed for 20 to 40 seconds until smooth and well combined.

3. Pour into a glass and serve immediately.

NUTRITION INFO Calories 139, Total Fat 0g, Carbohydrates 34g, Protein 3g, Cholesterol 0mg

> TIP To get as much juice as possible out of your lemon or lime, place it on a cutting board and roll it around gently for a few seconds using the palm of your hand. The combination of the warmth of your hand and the applied pressure will loosen the membranes that trap the juice inside the flesh.

Nutty Almond Butter–Banana Bites

SERVES I   PREP TIME: 5 MINUTES
MEAL PLAN ● ● ● ●

This recipe is incredibly easy to prepare and works well as both a breakfast dish and a snack. Feel free to swap out ingredients like chopped pecans or almonds for the walnuts. You can also try sprinkling your banana with a bit of ground cinnamon for extra flavor.

1 large green-tipped banana
2 tablespoons natural almond butter, divided
1 tablespoon finely chopped walnuts

1. Slice the banana in half lengthwise and spread 1 tablespoon of almond butter on each half.

2. Sprinkle with the walnuts and then cut the banana into 1-inch chunks and serve.

NUTRITION INFO Calories 349, Total Fat 21g, Carbohydrates 38g, Protein 10g, Cholesterol 0mg

Banana-Walnut Morning "Sundae"

SERVES 2   PREP TIME: 10 MINUTES
MEAL PLAN ● ● ● ● ●

This recipe is a delightfully indulgent way to start your morning. To prepare for this recipe the night before, place two cans of full-fat coconut milk upside down in the refrigerator before you go to bed. In the morning, the cream will have risen to the top, where you can easily spoon it off and whip it for the sundae.

> 2 (15-ounce) cans full-fat coconut milk, refrigerated upside down overnight
> ½ teaspoon ground cinnamon
> ¼ teaspoon ground nutmeg
> 1 cup sliced green-tipped banana
> ½ cup chopped raw walnuts

1. Turn the refrigerated cans of coconut milk right-side up and open them from the top.

2. Spoon the thick white paste into a large mixing bowl and beat on high speed with an electric mixer until stiff peaks form.

3. Beat in the cinnamon and nutmeg and then divide the coconut cream between two dishes.

4. Top the coconut cream with sliced banana, sprinkle with chopped walnuts, and serve.

NUTRITION INFO Calories 1,042, Total Fat 97g, Carbohydrates 35g, Protein 16g, Cholesterol 35mg

Breakfast Grains with Hazelnuts

**SERVES 2   PREP TIME: 15 MINUTES   COOK TIME: 20 MINUTES
MEAL PLAN** ● ○

Quinoa is a gluten-free, grain-like seed that is high in both dietary fiber and vegetarian protein. In this recipe, quinoa provides a hearty base for the dish as well as a number of important nutrients, including iron, lysine, and magnesium.

⅔ cup raw hazelnuts, toasted and chopped
1 tablespoon coconut oil
½ cup uncooked quinoa
1⅓ cups water
½ teaspoon coarse salt
2 teaspoons freshly grated ginger
1 teaspoon freshly grated lemon zest
2 tablespoons freshly squeezed lemon juice
⅓ cup plain Greek yogurt
Pinch ground nutmeg

1. In a large skillet, cook the hazelnuts over medium heat for 3 to 4 minutes, stirring often, until lightly browned. Set the nuts aside to cool.

2. In a medium saucepan, heat the coconut oil over medium-high heat. Add the quinoa and cook for 2 to 3 minutes, stirring often, until it is lightly toasted.

3. Pour in the water and add the salt, ginger, and lemon zest to the pan; stir well. Bring the water to a boil, then reduce the heat and simmer for 12 to 15 minutes until the grains are tender. Set aside to cool. ▶

4. In a medium mixing bowl, whisk together the lemon juice, yogurt, and nutmeg until smooth. Stir in the cooled grains and then fold in the toasted hazelnuts.

5. Spoon the mixture into two bowls and serve.

NUTRITION INFO Calories 390, Total Fat 25g, Carbohydrates 34g, Protein 11g, Cholesterol 13mg

Grain-Free Granola

SERVES 2 PREP TIME: 10 MINUTES COOK TIME: 15 MINUTES
MEAL PLAN ● ● ● ●

Nuts such as walnuts and almonds are rich in omega-3 fatty acids, which have been shown to help reduce blood cholesterol levels and improve heart health. Most nuts are also high in protein as well as other nutrients, including vitamin E, selenium, and iron. With this recipe you will benefit from a wide nutrient profile because it contains so many different kinds of nuts.

¼ cup raw hazelnuts

2 tablespoons raw walnut halves

2 tablespoons raw pecans

¼ cup raw almonds

2 tablespoons hulled sunflower seeds

2 tablespoons hulled pumpkin seeds

1 tablespoon ground flaxseed

¼ cup shredded unsweetened coconut

¼ teaspoon ground cinnamon

1 tablespoon coconut oil

1 teaspoon vanilla extract

¼ teaspoon coarse salt

1. Preheat the oven to 400°F.

2. In a large mixing bowl, combine the hazelnuts, walnuts, pecans, almonds, sunflower seeds, pumpkin seeds, flaxseed, coconut, and cinnamon, tossing well to combine.

3. In a small saucepan, whisk together the coconut oil, vanilla, and salt over medium heat until the oil is melted.

4. In the mixing bowl, toss the oil mixture with the granola until coated. Spread the mixture on a rimmed baking sheet and bake for 10 to 15 minutes, stirring every 5 minutes. ▶

5. Remove the baking sheet from the oven and allow the granola to cool before serving.

6. Store the granola in an airtight container.

NUTRITION INFO Calories 461, Total Fat 36g, Carbohydrates 23g, Protein 10g, Cholesterol 0mg

TIP The types and amounts of nuts and seeds listed in this recipe are just suggestions—feel free to make changes depending on your preferences. For example, you might omit the hazelnuts and double the walnuts, or use only pumpkin seeds rather than sunflower seeds. It's completely up to you!

Cheesy Bacon Breakfast Casserole

SERVES 2   PREP TIME: 10 MINUTES   COOK TIME: 20 MINUTES
MEAL PLAN ● ●

This cheesy breakfast casserole is the perfect dish to start your day. Feel free to customize your casserole by adding chopped yellow onion or garnishing it with sliced scallions. To enhance the presentation, sprinkle the casserole with some more shredded cheese during the last five minutes of baking time; if you add the cheese too much earlier, it could burn while cooking.

2 slices uncooked bacon, chopped
4 large eggs, lightly beaten
2 tablespoons whole milk
¼ teaspoon coarse salt
¼ teaspoon freshly ground black pepper
¼ cup shredded Cheddar cheese
Pinch ground cinnamon

1. Preheat the oven to 350°F.

2. In an oven-safe skillet, heat the bacon over medium-high heat. Cook until the bacon is crisp, stirring often, about 3 to 4 minutes.

3. In a large mixing bowl, whisk the eggs, milk, salt, and pepper until frothy. Add the cheese and cinnamon, and mix until well combined.

4. Add the egg mixture to the pan with the bacon and gently scramble for 2 to 3 minutes. ▶

5. Transfer to the oven and bake for 15 minutes until the egg is set.

6. Let it rest for 5 minutes before slicing to serve.

   NUTRITION INFO Calories 261, Total Fat 19g, Carbohydrates 2g, Protein 20g, Cholesterol 399mg

TIP To make this dish without the meat, you may choose to either omit the chopped bacon or replace it with diced mushrooms. Simply sauté the diced mushrooms in a bit of oil for 2 to 3 minutes before adding them to the casserole and transferring the dish to the oven.

Double-Boiler Scrambled Eggs

SERVES 2   PREP TIME: 5 MINUTES   COOK TIME: 10 MINUTES
MEAL PLAN ● ● ●

Cooking scrambled eggs slowly in a double boiler yields velvety eggs with a creamy texture that is unmatched by anything you can cook in a frying pan.

1 tablespoon coconut oil
4 large eggs, lightly beaten
2 tablespoons heavy cream
¼ teaspoon coarse salt

1. Fill a large saucepan with about 1 inch of water and set a large metal bowl or double boiler over the top of it, so the bottom of the bowl sits just above the water.

2. Heat the water to a simmer over medium-low heat and then pour the oil into the metal bowl or double boiler.

3. In a medium bowl, beat the eggs together with the heavy cream and salt, and pour the mixture into the double boiler once the oil has melted.

4. Cook the eggs until they just begin to firm up, 3 to 5 minutes, using a wooden spoon to gently scrape the eggs away from the sides of the double boiler as they cook.

5. Spoon the cooked eggs onto individual plates and serve hot.

NUTRITION INFO Calories 253, Total Fat 22g, Carbohydrates 1g, Protein 13g, Cholesterol 393mg

TIP If you're following the Blue meal plan, you can substitute unsweetened coconut milk for the heavy cream to make this recipe dairy-free. Making this substitution will also reduce the calorie and fat content of the recipe.

Egg and Prosciutto–Stuffed Mushroom Caps

SERVES 2   PREP TIME: 5 MINUTES   COOK TIME: 15 MINUTES
MEAL PLAN ● ● ●

In this recipe, portobello mushroom caps provide a tender base for egg and prosciutto. Portobello mushrooms also have the benefit of containing a number of important B vitamins as well as 15 percent of your daily value for potassium and nearly 25 percent of your daily value for copper.

2 large portobello mushroom caps
1 tablespoon extra-virgin olive oil
2 thin slices prosciutto
2 large eggs
Salt
Freshly ground black pepper
1 tablespoon chopped fresh basil
1 tablespoon chopped fresh parsley

1. Preheat the oven to 400°F.

2. Line a rimmed baking sheet with parchment paper and set it aside.

3. Clean the mushroom caps using a damp paper towel to remove any dirt. Use a sharp knife to cut the stems from the caps and to cut away the gills.

4. Brush the olive oil over the insides and outsides of the mushroom caps, and place them on the prepared baking sheet.

5. Fold a slice of prosciutto inside each mushroom cap and break an egg on top of each prosciutto slice, one per mushroom cap. Season with salt and pepper.

6. Bake for 10 to 15 minutes, until the egg is cooked through.

7. Remove the mushrooms from the oven and sprinkle them with the fresh herbs before serving.

    NUTRITION INFO Calories 225, Total Fat 16g, Carbohydrates 6g, Protein 16g, Cholesterol 211mg

TIP If you don't have any fresh herbs on hand, feel free to substitute dried basil and parsley. Keep in mind, however, that you will only need about 1 teaspoon of each rather than 2 tablespoons.

Crustless Spring Quiche

SERVES 2   PREP TIME: 5 MINUTES   COOK TIME: 15 MINUTES
MEAL PLAN ● ● ●

If you're cooking for two or a crowd and don't want to make an individual omelet for everyone, this crustless quiche is the perfect option. Simply combine the eggs and your favorite vegetables and bake it until the eggs are cooked through.

Cooking spray
4 large eggs, lightly beaten
1 tablespoon heavy cream
Salt
Freshly ground black pepper
1 cup frozen broccoli florets, thawed
¼ cup thinly sliced green bell pepper
2 tablespoons chopped fresh parsley
2 tablespoons chopped fresh cilantro

1. Preheat the oven to 350°F.

2. Coat a pie plate with cooking spray and set it aside.

3. In a medium mixing bowl, whisk together the eggs and cream until frothy, then season with salt and pepper.

4. Pour the mixture into the prepared pie plate and sprinkle in the broccoli and bell pepper.

5. Bake for 15 minutes or until the egg is set.

6. Remove the quiche from the oven, sprinkle the fresh herbs over the top, and serve immediately.

NUTRITION INFO Calories 189, Total Fat 13g, Carbohydrates 4g, Protein 14g, Cholesterol 382mg

Mexican Eggs

SERVES 2   PREP TIME: 5 MINUTES   COOK TIME: I5 MINUTES
MEAL PLAN ● ● ●

*This dish is the perfect combination of tender eggs and crunchy
vegetables, all cooked together and seasoned to perfection. It can be
customized according to your liking. If you prefer spicy food, add
another jalapeño pepper and a dash of cayenne pepper. If not, leave
out the jalapeño entirely.*

1 tablespoon extra-virgin olive oil
¼ cup diced yellow onion
½ cup diced tomato
½ jalapeño pepper, seeded and minced
1 teaspoon chopped fresh oregano
4 large eggs
Salt
Freshly ground black pepper
1 tablespoon chopped fresh cilantro
2 tablespoons shredded Cheddar cheese (optional)

1. In a large skillet, heat the oil over medium-high heat.

2. Stir in the onions and cook for 5 minutes or until just translucent. Add the tomatoes, jalapeño, and oregano and cook for
   3 minutes more, stirring often.

3. Push the vegetables to the side of the skillet and crack the
   eggs directly into the center. Season the eggs with salt and
   pepper and stir the mixture together, scrambling the eggs.

4. Cook for 3 to 4 minutes until the eggs are firm, then spoon the
   mixture onto individual dishes.

5. Garnish with the fresh cilantro and cheese (if using) to serve.

NUTRITION INFO Calories 247, Total Fat 19g, Carbohydrates 4g,
Protein 15g, Cholesterol 379mg

Poached Eggs with Tomato, Basil, and Avocado

SERVES 2   PREP TIME: 5 MINUTES   COOK TIME: 10 MINUTES
MEAL PLAN ● ○ ○ ●

In this recipe, the creamy texture of poached eggs pairs perfectly with the tomato and avocado, accented with a hint of fresh basil. The best part about this dish is that it's very easy to prepare—you can indulge in a fresh meal with a gourmet feel in only 10 minutes.

> 1 tablespoon distilled white vinegar
> 2 large eggs
> 2 thick slices fresh tomato
> 4 fresh basil leaves
> ½ ripe avocado, pitted and sliced
> Salt
> Freshly ground black pepper

1. Fill a medium skillet about two-thirds full with water and stir in the vinegar. Bring the mixture to a boil and then reduce the heat until it is just simmering.

2. Crack an egg over the skillet and gently drop it into the water. Use a spoon to gather the egg into a small mass, catching any tendrils that form in the water and scooping them in toward the egg.

3. Let the egg cook for 3 to 5 minutes until it is completely opaque, then remove it from the water using a slotted spoon.

4. Place the egg on a plate and cover it with a pot lid to keep warm.

5. Repeat steps 2 through 4 using the other egg.

6. Place a slice of tomato on each of two plates and top each one with two fresh basil leaves. Spoon a cooked egg on top of the basil, and top each serving with a few slices of avocado.

7. Season with salt and pepper before serving.

NUTRITION INFO Calories 179, Total Fat 15g, Carbohydrates 5g, Protein 7g, Cholesterol 186mg

SEVEN

MAKE-AHEAD SNACKS

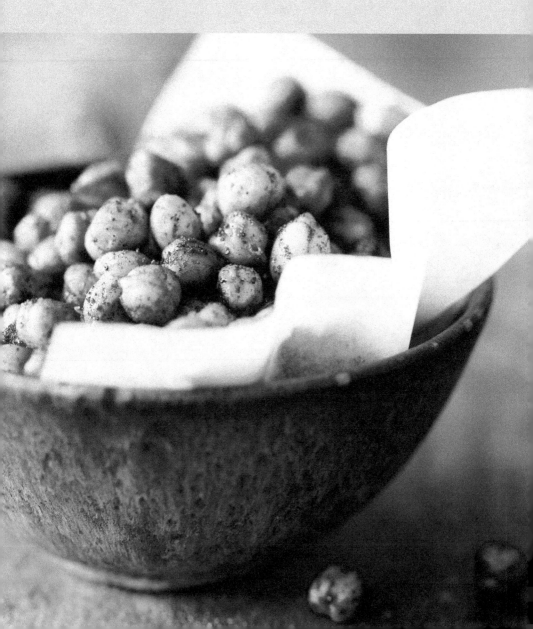

Spicy Roasted Chickpeas *92*

Crunchy Kale Chips *94*

Savory Couch Nuts *95*

Bacon-Wrapped Chicken Bites *96*

Homemade Hummus *97*

Lemon-Marinated Olives *98*

No-Mayo Deviled Eggs *99*

Cucumber and Tuna Salad Bites *100*

Roasted Edamame with Cracked Pepper *101*

Scallion Tofu Dip *102*

Roasted Eggplant Spread *103*

Jicama Salsa *104*

Baked Vegetable Chips *105*

Spicy Roasted Chickpeas

SERVES 4 TO 6   PREP TIME: 10 MINUTES   COOK TIME: 30 MINUTES
MEAL PLAN ● ●

Chickpeas, or garbanzo beans, are a versatile food that can be used in a variety of side dishes and salads. As you'll see in this recipe, however, they can also be a good snack food! These Spicy Roasted Chickpeas are great when you're in the mood for something crunchy with a bit of a kick. You may be surprised to find out just how easy it is to prepare these legumes—simply toss them in olive oil with your favorite spices and then roast them to perfection.

> 2 (15-ounce) cans chickpeas, drained and rinsed
> 3 tablespoons extra-virgin olive oil
> 1 tablespoon paprika
> 1 teaspoon cayenne pepper
> 1 teaspoon ground cumin
> 1 teaspoon coarse salt

1. Preheat the oven to 400°F.

2. Pat the chickpeas dry with a clean dish towel or paper towels.

3. In a large skillet, heat the oil over medium-high heat.

4. Stir in the paprika, cayenne pepper, cumin, and salt and cook for 30 seconds, stirring constantly.

5. Remove the skillet from the heat, then add the chickpeas to the skillet and toss them to coat with the oil.

6. Spread the chickpeas on a rimmed baking sheet and roast for 30 minutes, turning once halfway through.

7. Allow to cool to room temperature and serve. Store the leftovers in an airtight container.

NUTRITION INFO Calories 332, Total Fat 13.9g, Carbohydrates 37g, Protein 17g, Cholesterol 0mg

TIP Keep a close eye on the chickpeas as you roast them to make sure they don't burn. If you find that they're browning too quickly, reduce the oven temperature to 375°F and toss the chickpeas before returning them to the oven.

Crunchy Kale Chips

SERVES 3 TO 4   PREP TIME: 10 MINUTES   COOK TIME: 20 MINUTES
MEAL PLAN ● ● ● ●

When you're craving a crunchy snack, don't reach for that bag of potato chips! Potato chips are fried in oil and are often treated with all kinds of unnatural ingredients that can be bad for your health—this is not what you want to be putting into your body during a detox. If you want a salty, crunchy treat, then you definitely need to try these Crunchy Kale Chips. Baked kale has a nice crispy texture that will satisfy your urge to snack without putting you off track.

1 large head kale, torn into 2-inch chunks
3 tablespoons extra-virgin olive oil
1 teaspoon cayenne pepper
Coarse salt

1. Preheat the oven to 350°F.

2. Toss the kale with the oil and cayenne pepper, season with salt, then spread on a rimmed baking sheet in a single layer.

3. Bake for 20 minutes until crisp with lightly browned edges.

4. Remove from the oven and allow to cool before serving.

NUTRITION INFO Calories 188, Total Fat 14g, Carbohydrates 14g, Protein 4g, Cholesterol 0mg

Savory Couch Nuts

SERVES 4 TO 6   PREP TIME: 10 MINUTES   COOK TIME: 20 MINUTES
MEAL PLAN ● ○ ○ ○ ●

Nuts are the perfect snack food because they are full of protein and loaded with healthy nutrients. Plant sterols, a type of compound that exists naturally in nuts, have been shown to help improve cardio-vascular health and to reduce the risk for heart disease.

1 cup raw almonds

1 cup raw walnuts

1 cup raw pecans

1 cup shelled pistachios

⅓ cup extra-virgin olive oil

2 tablespoons vegetarian Worcestershire sauce

½ teaspoon ground cumin

Coarse salt to taste

1. Preheat the oven to 300°F.

2. In a large mixing bowl, combine the almonds, walnuts, pecans, and pistachios and toss with the olive oil, Worcestershire sauce, cumin, and salt.

3. Spread the mixture on a rimmed baking sheet and bake for 20 minutes, tossing once halfway through.

4. Remove from the oven and allow to cool before serving.

NUTRITION INFO Calories 765, Total Fat 72g, Carbohydrates 20g, Protein 20g, Cholesterol 0mg

TIP Worcestershire sauce is a fermented liquid often used to flavor meats. Because the sauce is made using anchovies, if you are following the Orange meal plan, you will need to find vegetarian Worcestershire sauce. You can also substitute an equal amount of coconut aminos, if you prefer.

Bacon-Wrapped Chicken Bites

SERVES 4   PREP TIME: 10 MINUTES   COOK TIME: 20 MINUTES
MEAL PLAN ◉ ◉ ●

These Bacon-Wrapped Chicken Bites are a meat lover's dream. Tender bites of boneless chicken wrapped in crispy bacon—what could be better? Enjoy them on their own or try dipping them in some gluten-free mustard or even the Green Goddess Dressing (page 211). Don't be afraid to experiment a bit when seasoning this dish—feel free to add a dash of cayenne pepper to give the bites a little kick or some mild chili powder for a burst of flavor. If you're worried about the salt content of your diet, don't add extra salt; you'll get plenty from the bacon.

1½ pounds boneless skinless chicken breast
1 pound thick-cut bacon, uncooked

1. Preheat the oven to 375°F.

2. Cut the chicken into 1-inch chunks and wrap each chunk in a half slice of bacon, using wooden toothpicks to keep the bacon in place.

3. Arrange the chicken bites on a parchment-lined baking sheet and bake for 20 minutes.

4. Transfer the chicken bites to a platter to serve.

NUTRITION INFO Calories 890, Total Fat 60g, Carbohydrates 0g, Protein 87g, Cholesterol 246mg

Homemade Hummus

SERVES 4 TO 6   PREP TIME: 5 MINUTES
MEAL PLAN ● ●

Hummus is a Middle Eastern dish made from chickpeas, or garbanzo beans. Traditionally, hummus is blended with tahini (a sauce made from sesame seeds) and olive oil with lemon juice and various spices added for flavor. Hummus is usually served with a drizzle of olive oil and a sprinkle of paprika in the middle. Keep in mind, however, that chickpeas are legumes, so this recipe is not approved for the Green or Blue meal plans.

2 (15-ounce) cans chickpeas
½ cup tahini
¼ cup extra-virgin olive oil
1 tablespoon minced garlic
1 tablespoon ground cumin
Juice of 1 lemon
Salt
Freshly ground black pepper
Paprika (optional)

1. Drain the chickpeas, reserving the liquid, then rinse them well.

2. In a food processor, combine the chickpeas with the tahini, oil, garlic, cumin, lemon juice, and reserved chickpea liquid. Season with salt and pepper. Blend until smooth and well combined.

3. Sprinkle with paprika (if using).

NUTRITION INFO Calories 529, Total Fat 32g, Carbohydrates 43g, Protein 22g, Cholesterol 0mg

TIP As you blend your hummus, keep an eye on its thickness and texture. If you find that it's too thick for your liking, add a little extra olive oil.

Lemon-Marinated Olives

SERVES 4 TO 6   PREP TIME: 10 MINUTES,
PLUS 30 MINUTES TO SOAK AND 2 DAYS TO MARINATE
MEAL PLAN ● ◌ ◌ ◌

The olive tree is native to the Mediterranean basin as well as parts of Africa, Asia, and China. The fruit of the tree is the olive, which can be eaten as is or pressed to extract olive oil, often used in cooking. These Lemon-Marinated Olives are perfect if you're seeking something with a salty flavor and a tender bite. Flavored with lemon juice and a hint of heat from the crushed red pepper flakes, they're one tasty snack.

1 pound large green olives
½ cup extra-virgin olive oil
1 tablespoon red wine vinegar
Juice and zest of 1 lemon
1 teaspoon crushed red pepper flakes
1 teaspoon minced garlic
½ teaspoon dried tarragon
½ teaspoon curry powder

1. Drain and rinse the olives, then soak them in cold water for at least 30 minutes.

2. Pour the olives into a colander to drain, and pat dry with a clean dish towel.

3. Toss the olives with the oil, vinegar, lemon juice and zest, red pepper flakes, garlic, tarragon, and curry powder. Transfer to a glass jar.

4. Cover the jar tightly with the lid and store at room temperature for at least 2 days before serving.

NUTRITION INFO Calories 409, Total Fat 44g, Carbohydrates 8g, Protein 1g, Cholesterol 0mg

No-Mayo Deviled Eggs

SERVES 2   PREP TIME: 15 MINUTES
MEAL PLAN ● ○ ○ ●

Many people who don't like deviled eggs say it's because they don't like mayonnaise. If this is the case for you, or if you're simply curious about a new deviled egg recipe, these No-Mayo Deviled Eggs will fill the bill. A single tablespoon of olive oil helps give the mashed egg yolks a creamy consistency, while mustard powder and Worcestershire sauce provide a hint of flavor. These deviled eggs are sure to be a hit at your next dinner party or family gathering.

8 hardboiled eggs, peeled
1 teaspoon distilled white vinegar
1 tablespoon extra-virgin olive oil
¼ teaspoon mustard powder
1 teaspoon vegetarian Worcestershire sauce
¼ teaspoon coarse salt
¼ teaspoon freshly ground black pepper
¼ teaspoon paprika

1. Cut the eggs in half and carefully transfer the yolks to a medium mixing bowl.

2. Mash the yolks with a fork, then stir in the vinegar, oil, mustard powder, Worcestershire sauce, salt, and pepper until a creamy mixture forms.

3. Arrange the egg whites on a serving dish and spoon the filling back into the centers.

4. Garnish with paprika to serve.

NUTRITION INFO Calories 316, Total Fat 25g, Carbohydrates 2g, Protein 22g, Cholesterol 655mg

Cucumber and Tuna Salad Bites

SERVES 4 TO 6   PREP TIME: I5 MINUTES
MEAL PLAN ● ○ ●

This filling snack or lunch is a pleasing blend of crunchy and creamy. Its foundation is a hollowed-out cucumber, which provides the crunch, while the filling is a type of tuna salad that has a cool and creamy texture. If you can't finish the whole dish at once, use only half the cucumber and wrap the other half in plastic wrap, then store it in the refrigerator. This will keep it fresh for when you're ready to use it—simply unwrap it and slice to serve.

1 large English cucumber, peeled
1 (6-ounce) can tuna in water, drained
1 tablespoon freshly squeezed lemon juice
¼ cup finely diced celery
2 tablespoons Mayonnaise (page 206)
2 tablespoons chopped fresh basil
Salt
Freshly ground black pepper

1. Cut the cucumber in half lengthwise and use a small knife to hollow out the center.

2. In a medium mixing bowl, flake the tuna and toss with the lemon juice, celery, Mayonnaise, and basil. Season with salt and pepper.

3. Spoon the tuna mixture into the cucumbers.

4. Slice the cucumbers into 1-inch chunks and arrange on a platter to serve.

NUTRITION INFO Calories 97, Total Fat 4g, Carbohydrates 5g, Protein 11g, Cholesterol 20mg

Roasted Edamame with Cracked Pepper

SERVES 2   PREP TIME: 5 MINUTES   COOK TIME: 30 MINUTES
MEAL PLAN ● ○

Edamame is simply a preparation method used for immature soybean pods. This food is popular in Taiwanese, Chinese, and Japanese cuisine and is catching on in the United States. The name edamame *is derived from the Japanese for "twig bean," which is a fairly accurate description of what the bean looks like. Edamame is a crunchy, tasty snack that is low in calories and high in nutrients. A 100-gram serving contains nearly 80 percent of your daily value for folate and almost 50 percent of your daily value for manganese, not to mention plenty of vitamin K, iron, and magnesium.*

½ pound frozen shelled edamame

1 teaspoon extra-virgin olive oil

¾ teaspoon coarse salt

½ teaspoon freshly ground black pepper

1. Preheat the oven to 375°F.

2. Let the edamame thaw completely, then pat dry with a clean dish towel.

3. In a mixing bowl, toss the edamame with the olive oil, salt, and pepper, then spread on a rimmed baking sheet in a single layer.

4. Roast for 30 minutes, turning every 5 minutes or so, until lightly browned all over.

5. Allow to cool before serving.

NUTRITION INFO Calories 165, Total Fat 8g, Carbohydrates 11g, Protein 12g, Cholesterol 0mg

Scallion Tofu Dip

SERVES 4   PREP TIME: 5 MINUTES
MEAL PLAN ● ●

If you like to snack, then this Scallion Tofu Dip is one recipe you'll definitely want to keep on hand. Whip up a big batch of it and keep it in the fridge for when you need a quick bite between meals. This dip pairs perfectly with fresh carrots and celery, or you can use it as a topping for cooked chicken and fish. In addition to being full of delicious flavor, this recipe is also packed with nutrients. From the tofu you get plenty of vegetarian protein, and the spinach delivers vitamin K, vitamin C, and manganese.

1 (10-ounce) bag frozen spinach, thawed

4 ounces silken tofu, chopped

2 scallions, sliced

2 tablespoons freshly squeezed lemon juice

1 tablespoon coconut aminos or tamari

1 teaspoon minced garlic

1 teaspoon cayenne pepper

1. Squeeze as much moisture from the spinach as possible and place it in a food processor.

2. Add the tofu, scallions, lemon juice, coconut aminos, garlic, and cayenne pepper, and blend until smooth and well combined.

3. Spoon the dip into a bowl and serve with sliced vegetables for dipping.

NUTRITION INFO Calories 42, Total Fat 1g, Carbohydrates 5g, Protein 4g, Cholesterol 0mg

TIP For this recipe it's especially important that you use tofu with a soft texture—silken tofu is the best. Firm or extra-firm tofu will not provide the creamy texture you need for this dip.

Roasted Eggplant Spread

SERVES 4   PREP TIME: 10 MINUTES   COOK TIME: 20 MINUTES
MEAL PLAN ● ○ ○ ●

*This guilt-free dip is so tasty and satisfying that it's hard to believe
how low it is in calories. Try it with carrot sticks, celery, or the Crunchy
Kale Chips recipe (page 94). Make a large batch and store it in the
refrigerator for up to five days.*

1 large eggplant, peeled and diced
1 garlic clove, peeled
1 large green bell pepper, diced
1 jalapeño pepper
½ yellow onion, roughly chopped
2 tablespoons extra-virgin olive oil
Salt
Freshly ground black pepper
1 cup fresh basil leaves

1. Preheat the oven to 425°F.

2. On a large sheet pan, place the prepared eggplant, garlic, bell
   pepper, jalapeño pepper, and onion.

3. Drizzle the pan with the olive oil and season with the salt
   and pepper.

4. Roast for 20 minutes, turning once until the vegetables are
   slightly golden and tender. Set aside to cool slightly.

5. Transfer the mixture to a food processor fitted with a steel
   blade, and add the basil. Pulse until well mixed.

6. Serve at room temperature or refrigerate.

   NUTRITION INFO Calories 111, Total Fat 7g, Carbohydrates 11g,
   Protein 2g, Cholesterol 0mg

Jicama Salsa

SERVES 2 PREP TIME: I0 MINUTES
MEAL PLAN ● ● ● ●

Sweet and crunchy jicama makes for a fun and fresh snack. One cup has only 46 calories but 6 grams of tummy-pleasing fiber. Eat this salsa by the spoonful or serve with gluten-free chips or crackers for dipping. You can chop all the ingredients by hand, but using a food processor saves a ton of time.

1 large jicama, peeled and diced
½ bell pepper, diced
½ cup fresh cilantro
¼ yellow onion
Juice of one lime
Coarse salt

1. Put the jicama, bell pepper, cilantro, and onion in a food processor fitted with a steel blade.

2. Season with the lime juice and salt.

3. Pulse until the ingredients are well chopped.

4. Serve with gluten-free chips or crackers.

NUTRITION INFO Calories 244, Total Fat 1g, Carbohydrates 51g, Protein 5g, Cholesterol 0mg

Baked Vegetable Chips

SERVES 2   PREP TIME: 5 MINUTES   COOK TIME: 20 MINUTES
MEAL PLAN ●○○○

These veggie chips taste better than anything out of a bag. Experiment with various veggies and find your favorite flavor combination. For best results, use a mandoline for even and extra thin slices.

> 1 bulb fennel, thinly sliced
> 1 sweet potato, peeled and thinly sliced
> 2 parsnips, thinly sliced
> 1 tablespoon extra-virgin olive oil

1. Preheat the oven to 400°F.

2. Place the fennel, sweet potato, and parsnip slices on a sheet pan.

3. Drizzle with the olive oil and season with the salt and pepper.

4. Toss gently to coat.

5. Bake until crisp, about 20 minutes.

6. Serve as is or with one of the salsa or dip recipes in this book.

NUTRITION INFO Calories 248, Total Fat 8g, Carbohydrates 44g, Protein 4g, Cholesterol 0mg

EIGHT

SALADS, SOUPS, SANDWICHES & SIDES

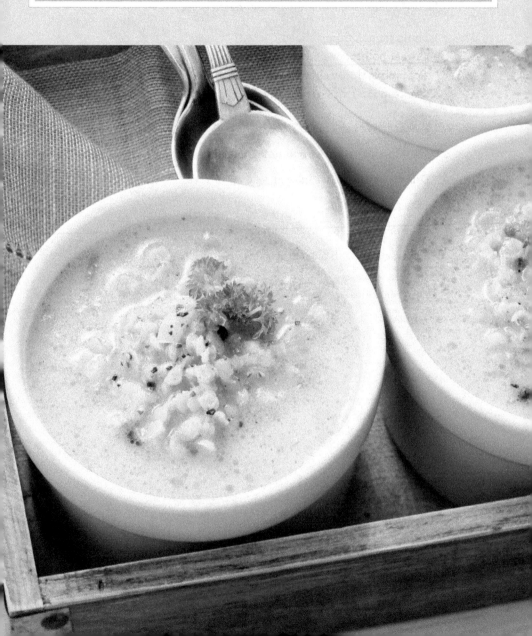

Bacon and Broccoli Salad *108*

Chicken Salad with Walnuts *109*

Balsamic Quinoa-Spinach Salad *110*

Steak Salad with Goat Cheese *112*

Guacamole Salad with Chicken *114*

Arugula and White Bean Salad *115*

Asparagus and Prosciutto Salad *116*

Slow-Cooked Creamy Black Beans *117*

Hummus, Cheese, and Avocado Tostadas *118*

Sweet Pea Soup *119*

Pumpkin-Sage Soup *120*

Curried Carrot Soup with Basil *121*

Quick Curried Lentil Stew *122*

Eggplant Sandwiches with Herbed Feta *124*

Bacon and Broccoli Salad

SERVES | PREP TIME: 10 MINUTES
MEAL PLAN ● ●

This salad offers the perfect combination of crunchy broccoli, crispy bacon, and creamy dressing. If you're looking for a side dish to pair with your favorite grilled chicken or fish, this is a great option. Even after you complete your sugar detox, you may find yourself continuing to make this recipe simply because it works so well to accompany everything from picnic foods to family dinners at home. The key is to use fresh broccoli so it's crisp and flavorful.

2 cups broccoli florets, chopped into bite-size chunks
¼ cup shredded Cheddar cheese
1 tablespoon toasted sunflower seeds
1 tablespoon toasted pumpkin seeds
2 tablespoons Mayonnaise (page 206)
Salt
Freshly ground black pepper
1 strip cooked bacon, crumbled

1. In a large bowl, stir together the broccoli, cheese, and toasted sunflower and pumpkin seeds.

2. Toss with the Mayonnaise and season with the salt and pepper.

3. Sprinkle the crumbled bacon on top to serve.

NUTRITION INFO Calories 389, Total Fat 28g, Carbohydrates 22g, Protein 17g, Cholesterol 42mg

TIP When you're preparing the broccoli for this recipe, don't be afraid to use the entire stalk—don't stop with just the florets. Because you are chopping the broccoli into bite-size pieces, it doesn't matter whether they come from the head or the stalk.

Chicken Salad with Walnuts

SERVES 2   PREP TIME: 10 MINUTES
MEAL PLAN

This recipe provides the perfect opportunity to use the leftovers from your Lemon-Thyme Roasted Chicken (page 174). Simply remove any skin and bones from the chicken and chop it into bite-size pieces. You can use both white and dark meat for this recipe or whichever you prefer. The tender, lemon-seasoned chicken will blend perfectly with crunchy walnuts to produce a cool, satisfying salad that the whole family will love for lunch, dinner, or an afternoon snack.

2 cups cooked boneless skinless chicken breast, chopped
½ cup thinly sliced celery
½ cup chopped walnuts
1 tablespoon chopped fresh dill
¼ cup plain Greek yogurt
Juice of ½ lemon
Salt
Freshly ground black pepper

1. In a large mixing bowl, stir together the chicken, celery, walnuts, and dill.

2. Toss with the yogurt and lemon juice, then season with the salt and pepper.

NUTRITION INFO Calories 495, Total Fat 31g, Carbohydrates 7g, Protein 50g, Cholesterol 131mg

Balsamic Quinoa-Spinach Salad

SERVES 2   PREP TIME: 10 MINUTES   COOK TIME: 15 MINUTES

MEAL PLAN ● ◐

This recipe is halfway between a side dish and a salad because it contains elements of both. Fresh baby spinach provides a salad base while tender quinoa lends a bit of weight to the dish. Top it all off with balsamic dressing and a handful of sliced scallions, and you have the perfect spring or summer meal. If you don't plan to eat all of this salad at once, don't add the balsamic vinegar and olive oil to the entire salad—dress only the part you intend to eat so it doesn't get soggy in the refrigerator. Save even more time by making the quinoa the night before.

⅓ cup uncooked quinoa
⅔ cups vegetable broth
3 cups fresh baby spinach leaves, packed
½ cup diced tomatoes
2 tablespoons hulled pumpkin seeds
1 scallion, sliced thin
2 tablespoons balsamic vinegar
1 tablespoon extra-virgin olive oil
Salt
Freshly ground black pepper

1. In a small saucepan, stir together the quinoa and broth and bring to a boil.

2. Reduce the heat and simmer, covered, for 15 minutes, until the quinoa absorbs the liquid.

3. Turn off the heat and let stand, covered, for 5 minutes while you prepare the salad.

4. In a large salad bowl, toss together the spinach, tomatoes, pumpkin seeds, and scallions.

5. Add the cooked quinoa, balsamic vinegar, and oil. Season with salt and pepper. Toss to combine.

6. Chill until ready to serve.

NUTRITION INFO Calories 279, Total Fat 10g, Carbohydrates 36g, Protein 8g, Cholesterol 0mg

TIP Using broth instead of water makes the quinoa more flavorful. To enhance the flavor even more, consider toasting it before cooking. To do so, simply heat the rinsed quinoa in a dry skillet over medium heat until it begins to brown. Then just add your broth and boil the quinoa as directed.

Steak Salad with Goat Cheese

SERVES 2 PREP TIME: 10 MINUTES
MEAL PLAN

Here's a great way to use your leftovers from your Argentinean-Style Beef (page 181). This salad changes dramatically in flavor based on the kind of cheese you use, as well as the addition of new ingredients, such as avocado, carrot, marinated artichoke hearts, chopped tomatoes, asparagus, broccoli florets, watercress, spinach, baby arugula, or kale. Experiment with different combinations and the various dressings in this book and find your favorite. If you think that a salad has to be boring or unsatisfying, this recipe will make you reconsider!

¼ cup pumpkin seeds
6 cups romaine lettuce, cut into bite-size pieces
¾ cup canned hearts of palm, drained and chopped
½ medium cucumber, diced
¼ medium red onion, sliced into rings
2 ounces goat cheese, crumbled
4 ounces cooked beef, sliced into strips
1 recipe Green Goddess Dressing (page 211)

1. In a small skillet, cook the pumpkin seeds over medium heat for 2 to 3 minutes, stirring often, until lightly browned. Set the seeds aside to cool.

2. In a large salad bowl, toss together the lettuce, hearts of palm, and cucumber.

3. Top the salad with the red onion and sprinkle the goat cheese on top.

4. Place the sliced steak on top of the salad and sprinkle with the toasted pumpkin seeds.

5. Serve the salad with the Green Goddess Dressing on the side.

NUTRITION INFO Calories 447, Total Fat 29g, Carbohydrates 16g, Protein 33g, Cholesterol 83mg

TIP When it comes to buying goat cheese, you have many options to choose from. Brunet is a soft-ripened cheese with a silky texture like that of whipped cream—it has subtle notes of mushroom and sweet cream flavor. Garrotxa is semi-firm with an herby hazelnut flavor. Crottin de Chavignol is a drier cheese with an intense flavor.

Guacamole Salad with Chicken

SERVES I   PREP TIME: 10 MINUTES
MEAL PLAN ● ◦ ●

Nachos are a popular, tempting choice for movie or game night. Loaded with protein and healthy fats, this salad has way more flavor than a dish of greasy nachos. Creamy avocado helps dress the veggies, and lean chicken makes this a satisfying meal.

3 cups mixed greens
1 cup chopped tomato
½ avocado, diced
1 tablespoon chopped fresh cilantro
1 tablespoon extra-virgin olive oil
Juice of ½ lime
4 ounces grilled or roasted chicken breast
Crushed, baked gluten-free tortilla chips for garnish

1. In a large salad bowl, toss together the greens, tomato, avocado, cilantro, oil, and lime juice.

2. Top with the chicken and tortilla chips and serve.

NUTRITION INFO Calories 758, Total Fat 51g, Carbohydrates 33g, Protein 51g, Cholesterol 97mg

Arugula and White Bean Salad

A hearty and satisfying salad does not have to contain meat. Protein from the beans and high-fiber vegetables in this dish will keep you feeling satisfied all afternoon long. Arugula is filled with nutrients including vitamins A, C, and K, iron, potassium, and copper.

2 tablespoons extra-virgin olive oil

2 teaspoons balsamic vinegar

Salt

Freshly ground black pepper

3 cups fresh arugula

½ medium cucumber, sliced

¼ cup thinly sliced red onion

½ cup canned cannellini beans, rinsed and drained

1. In a large bowl, combine the oil and vinegar.

2. Season with the salt and pepper and whisk well.

3. Add the arugula, cucumber, red onion, and beans.

4. Toss well and serve immediately.

NUTRITION INFO Calories 599, Total Fat 29g, Carbohydrates 66g, Protein 24g, Cholesterol 0mg

Asparagus and Prosciutto Salad

A classic combination of fresh veggies, finished with a touch of salty prosciutto and a drizzle of tangy balsamic vinegar, this salad is sure to satisfy. Asparagus is an excellent source of many nutrients, including vitamins A, C, E, and K. To steam the asparagus, microwave it with a small amount of water for 2 minutes until fork tender but still crisp.

3 cups mixed greens
Coarse salt
Freshly ground black pepper
6 to 8 large asparagus spears, trimmed and chopped
1 cup sliced cucumber
1 tablespoon balsamic vinegar
Extra-virgin olive oil, for drizzling
3 thin slices prosciutto, roughly chopped or torn
2 tablespoons grated or shredded Parmesan cheese

1. Put the greens in a large bowl and season with the salt and pepper.

2. Top the greens with the asparagus and cucumber.

3. Drizzle with the vinegar and oil and toss well to coat.

4. Top with the prosciutto and cheese and serve.

NUTRITION INFO Calories 340, Total Fat 25g, Carbohydrates 16g, Protein 20g, Cholesterol 45mg

Slow-Cooked Creamy Black Beans

**SERVES 2 TO 4   PREP TIME: 5 MINUTES   COOK TIME: 10 MINUTES,
PLUS 2 HOURS TO SIMMER (SEE TIP)
MEAL PLAN** ● ●

*In addition to their delicious flavor and tender texture, black beans
are known for their high protein content. They also contain a variety of
nutrients including molybdenum, folate, fiber, manganese, and copper.*

2 cups dried black beans
Water
1 large garlic clove, smashed
½ teaspoon ground cumin
1 bay leaf
Salt
Freshly ground black pepper

1. Rinse the beans well in cool water and pick through them to
   discard any small stones.

2. Soak the beans in water overnight, then drain well.

3. Place the beans in a 3½- or 5-quart slow cooker along with the
   garlic, cumin, and bay leaf.

4. Add enough water to cover the beans by about 2 inches and
   stir to combine.

5. Cover and cook on low for 6 to 8 hours.

6. When the beans are tender, season with the salt and pepper
   and serve hot.

NUTRITION INFO Calories 524, Total Fat 2g, Carbohydrates 97g,
Protein 32g, Cholesterol 0mg

TIP If you're pressed for time, make this recipe with 2 (15-ounce)
cans of black beans.

Hummus, Cheese, and Avocado Tostadas

SERVES 2   PREP TIME: IO MINUTES   COOK TIME: 5 MINUTES
MEAL PLAN ● ●

*This dish is a Mexican delight for pizza lovers but free of gluten
and packed with protein. Use black beans instead of hummus for a
different flavor and texture option. Serve with a side salad for a
complete meal.*

4 corn tortillas
4 tablespoons prepared hummus
½ cup Cheddar cheese, shredded
¼ cup chopped fresh cilantro
1 avocado, diced

1. Preheat the broiler.

2. Arrange the tortillas in an even layer on the baking sheet.
   Spread with the hummus and top with the shredded cheese.

3. Broil for 2 to 3 minutes, or until the cheese is melted.

4. Serve topped with the cilantro and diced avocado.

NUTRITION INFO Calories 477, Total Fat 33g, Carbohydrates 37g,
Protein 13g, Cholesterol 30mg

Sweet Pea Soup

SERVES 2   PREP TIME: 5 MINUTES   COOK TIME: 10 MINUTES
MEAL PLAN ● ●

This is quite possibly the easiest soup you'll ever make! Peas are an amazing source of protein, fiber, iron, and antioxidants. A quick simmer and whirl from the blender, and a nutrition-packed lunch is served.

2 cups fresh or frozen (thawed) green peas
2 cups vegetable broth
Sea salt
Red pepper flakes (optional)
Extra-virgin olive oil, for drizzling

1. In a medium saucepan, bring the peas and broth to a simmer.

2. Using an immersion blender, puree until smooth.

3. Season with salt and red pepper (if using) and drizzle with the olive oil before serving.

NUTRITION INFO Calories 183, Total Fat 4g, Carbohydrates 24g, Protein 13g, Cholesterol 0mg

Pumpkin-Sage Soup

SERVES 2 TO 4   PREP TIME: 10 MINUTES   COOK TIME: 20 MINUTES
MEAL PLAN ● ● ● ●

This winter squash is not just for the holidays. Look for 100 percent real canned pumpkin, not pumpkin pie filling that is loaded with sugar. Coconut milk makes this soup extra smooth and velvety, but there is no dairy to be found. If you prefer a blended soup, puree with an immersion blender before serving.

> 1 tablespoon coconut oil
> ½ medium yellow onion, chopped
> 3 tablespoons chopped fresh sage
> Salt
> Freshly ground black pepper
> 1 (15-ounce) can pumpkin puree
> 2 cups vegetable broth
> 1 (15 ounce) can coconut milk

1. In a large soup pot, heat the oil.

2. Add the onion and the sage. Season with the salt and pepper, and sauté for 5 minutes, until the onion is tender.

3. Add the pumpkin puree, vegetable broth, and coconut milk; stir well to combine.

4. Taste for seasoning and then add more salt and pepper, if desired.

5. Bring to a boil, stirring well.

6. Reduce the heat to a simmer and cook for an additional 15 minutes, until warmed through, and serve.

NUTRITION INFO Calories 696, Total Fat 59g, Carbohydrates 37g, Protein 14g, Cholesterol 0mg

Curried Carrot Soup with Basil

SERVES 2 TO 3 PREP TIME: 10 MINUTES   COOK TIME: 20 MINUTES
MEAL PLAN ● ● ● ●

Warm up on a cool winter evening with this fast-cooking soup. Believe it or not, frozen vegetables are just as nutritious as fresh, and for this recipe, they are a huge time-saver. This soup is overflowing with antioxidants like beta-carotene, and the spices in the curry powder offer additional anti-inflammatory properties.

1 tablespoon extra-virgin olive oil
½ medium yellow onion, chopped
1 garlic clove, minced
1 tablespoon curry powder
½ teaspoon coarse salt
3 cups vegetable broth
1 (16 ounce) bag frozen carrots
½ cup fresh basil leaves

1. In a medium soup pot, heat the oil.

2. Add the onion, garlic, and curry powder. Season with the salt and cook for 5 minutes. Add the vegetable broth and carrots and stir.

3. Bring mixture to a boil, then reduce the heat to a simmer and cook for 15 minutes, stirring occasionally, until carrots are very tender.

4. Turn off the heat and stir in the basil.

5. Puree using an immersion blender or carefully transfer the mixture to a blender in batches.

6. Blend until smooth and serve.

NUTRITION INFO Calories 236, Total Fat 10g, Carbohydrates 29g, Protein 10g, Cholesterol 0mg

Quick Curried Lentil Stew

SERVES 2   PREP TIME: 10 MINUTES   COOK TIME: 20 MINUTES
MEAL PLAN ● ●

If you're looking for a hot and hearty recipe that is easy to prepare, look no further than this stew. Not only are lentils known for their high protein content, but they also have a creamy texture that works well in stews like this one. Canned coconut milk adds to the pleasant consistency of this dish. Don't make the mistake of using unsweetened coconut milk from a carton—only full-fat coconut milk will give this dish the thickness that it requires to be called a stew.

2 tablespoons extra-virgin olive oil, divided
½ medium yellow onions, chopped
1 medium carrot, peeled and chopped
1 cup water
1 (15-ounce) can yellow lentils, rinsed and drained
1 cup canned full-fat coconut milk
¼ cup unsweetened shredded coconut
¼ teaspoon coarse salt
1 bay leaf
1 teaspoon minced garlic
¼ teaspoon ground ginger
½ teaspoon curry powder
Sprigs of fresh parsley, for garnish

1. In a large skillet over medium heat, heat 1 tablespoon of oil.

2. Add the onions and carrot and cook for 5 to 6 minutes, stirring often, until caramelized.

3. Stir in the water, lentils, coconut milk, coconut, salt, and bay leaf, then bring to a boil.

4. Reduce the heat and simmer, uncovered, for 10 minutes to allow the stew to thicken.

5. Meanwhile, in a small saucepan, heat the remaining 1 table-spoon of oil over medium heat. Add the garlic, ginger, and curry powder, and cook for 2 minutes, stirring often.

6. Stir the curry mixture into the soup, then remove the bay leaf. Remove the pan from the heat.

7. Using an immersion blender, puree the soup until smooth.

8. Serve hot, garnished with fresh sprigs of parsley.

NUTRITION INFO Calories 594, Total Fat 51g, Carbohydrates 29g, Protein 6g, Cholesterol 10mg

Eggplant Sandwiches with Herbed Feta

SERVES 2   PREP TIME: 10 MINUTES   COOK TIME: 15 MINUTES
MEAL PLAN ● ○ ○

Who says a sandwich has to be served on bread? These Eggplant Sandwiches with Herbed Feta are everything a sandwich should be, with no grains whatsoever. Even more amazing is the fact that this dish is so easy to prepare. Simply sauté the eggplant slices in a little olive oil and layer them on either side of a dollop of herbed feta cheese. If you're feeling adventurous, you might even try substituting goat cheese or another soft white cheese for the feta. The options are endless if you use your imagination! For extra fast preparation, cook the eggplant slices ahead and store in the fridge. Reheat in the microwave or a nonstick skillet.

2 ounces feta cheese
1 garlic clove, minced
1 tablespoon chopped fresh parsley
1 tablespoon chopped fresh basil
1 tablespoon extra-virgin olive oil
Coconut oil, for cooking
1 small eggplant, peeled and sliced 1 inch thick
Coarse salt

1. In a medium mixing bowl, stir the feta, garlic, parsley, basil, and olive oil until creamy and well combined. Set aside.

2. In a large skillet, heat a few teaspoons of coconut oil over medium-high heat.

3. Blot the eggplant slices dry with a paper towel. Season with salt on both sides, then add to the hot skillet.

4. Cook the slices for 5 to 6 minutes on each side, until heated through but not soft.

5. Place one eggplant slice on each of four plates and top each with a tablespoon or so of the feta mixture.

6. Top each with another slice of eggplant and serve the sandwiches hot.

NUTRITION INFO Calories 215, Total Fat 16g, Carbohydrates 15g, Protein 7g, Cholesterol 25mg

NINE

VEGETARIAN MAINS

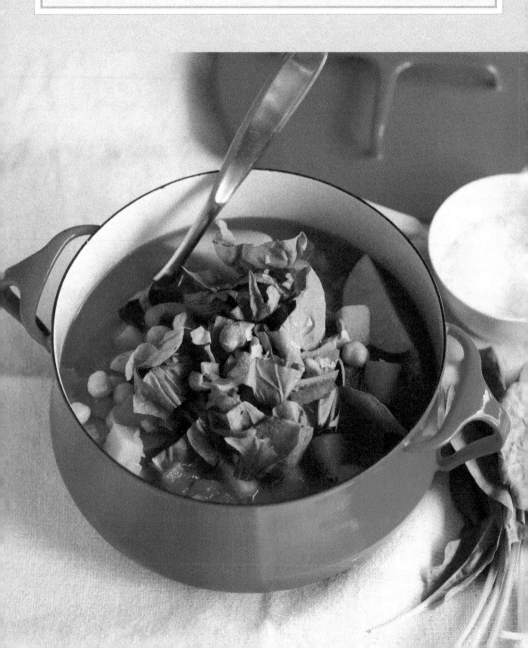

Grilled Portobello Mushrooms
with Whipped Parsnips *128*

Lemon and Arugula Pasta *130*

Spinach and Feta Summer Squash "Pasta" *132*

Ricotta-Stuffed Spaghetti Squash *134*

Lentil–Brown Rice Casserole *136*

Spiced Chickpeas with Grilled Tofu *137*

Asian Slaw with Thai Tofu *139*

Sesame-Ginger Soba Noodles *141*

Quinoa Tabblouleh *142*

Ratatouille *144*

Ratatouille-Stuffed Peppers *146*

Tempeh and Swiss Chard Stir-Fry *147*

Spinach and White Bean Stew *148*

Quinoa Cakes *150*

White Chili *152*

Grilled Portobello Mushrooms with Whipped Parsnips

SERVES 2   PREP TIME: 5 MINUTES   COOK TIME: 20 MINUTES
MEAL PLAN ● ● ●

Parsnips are a type of root vegetable known for their naturally sweet flavor that is divine when paired with earthy mushrooms. Though in this recipe whipped parsnips may look like potatoes, they are actually closely related to the carrot. Parsnips produce long, fleshy roots that are larger and sweeter than carrots, but they are white in color rather than orange. They are incredibly rich in dietary fiber, which helps improve digestion and reduce blood cholesterol levels. They're packed with polyacetylene, an antioxidant that may help prevent certain types of cancer.

FOR THE MUSHROOMS

4 large portobello mushroom caps
1 tablespoon extra-virgin olive oil
1 tablespoon balsamic vinegar
Salt
Freshly ground black pepper

FOR THE WHIPPED PARSNIPS

8 ounces parsnips, peeled and chopped in to ½-inch pieces
¼ cup heavy cream
1 tablespoon coconut oil
½ teaspoon ground nutmeg
Salt
Freshly ground black pepper

To make the mushrooms

1. Heat a grill or grill pan over medium-high heat.

2. Remove the stems from the mushrooms and, using a spoon, clean out the dark brown gills from the underside of the caps; set aside.

3. In a small bowl, whisk together the olive oil and vinegar.

4. Drizzle both sides of the mushrooms with the vinegar mixture and season well with salt and pepper.

5. Grill for 3 minutes per side, until tender. Thinly slice before serving with parsnips.

To make the whipped parsnips

1. Bring a large pot of salted water to a boil and add the parsnips.

2. Cook the parsnips until very tender, about 15 minutes, then drain, reserving ½ cup of the cooking liquid.

3. Return the parsnips to the pot and stir in the cream, oil, and nutmeg.

4. Beat the parsnips with an electric hand mixer until smooth and creamy, adding some of the reserved cooking liquid if needed to thin them.

5. Season with salt and pepper and serve hot.

NUTRITION INFO Calories 305, Total Fat 20g, Carbohydrates 30g, Protein 6g, Cholesterol 21mg

Lemon and Arugula Pasta

SERVES 2 PREP TIME: 5 MINUTES COOK TIME: 20 MINUTES
MEAL PLAN ● ○

Also known as rocket, arugula is an incredibly healthy vegetable that offers significant detoxification benefits. It contains more than eight times the calcium content and five times the vitamin A and C content of iceberg lettuce and is also rich in iron and vitamin K. In this recipe, arugula may seem like an afterthought or an add-on, but the reality is that it is the star of the dish. To make the most of this recipe, buy fresh arugula and rinse it well to minimize the bitterness.

4 ounces gluten-free pasta
2 tablespoons extra-virgin olive oil, divided
1 garlic clove, minced
Pinch crushed red pepper flakes
1 cup diced tomato
3 cups fresh arugula, rinsed well
Zest and juice of one lemon
¼ teaspoon coarse salt
½ teaspoon freshly ground black pepper
¼ cup grated Parmesan cheese

1. Bring a large pot of salted water to a boil and add the gluten-free pasta.

2. Cook the pasta for 10 to 12 minutes, until bite-tender, according to the directions. Drain and set aside.

3. In a large skillet, heat 1 tablespoon of oil over medium-high heat.

4. Stir in the garlic and red pepper flakes and cook for 30 seconds. Add the tomato, arugula, and lemon zest and cook for 2 minutes, until the arugula is wilted.

5. Stir in the cooked pasta along with the remaining 1 tablespoon of oil, lemon juice, salt, and pepper. Toss well and cook until heated through.

6. Garnish with fresh Parmesan to serve.

NUTRITION INFO Calories 449, Total Fat 22g, Carbohydrates 47g, Protein 18g, Cholesterol 20mg

TIP Gluten-free pasta cooks differently from traditional pasta, and it's all too easy to overcook it. Follow package directions but make sure to test the pasta regularly to make sure that it doesn't become mushy before you remove the pot from the stove.

Spinach and Feta Summer Squash "Pasta"

SERVES 2   PREP TIME: 15 MINUTES   COOK TIME: 25 MINUTES
MEAL PLAN ● ●

Tasty summer squash substitutes for traditional pasta in this delicious Italian-style dish. The squash gives the sauce something to cling to, and it should satisfy your desire for pasta during this detox. If you don't like feta cheese, you can substitute any hard Italian cheese, such as Parmesan, Asiago, or Romano cheeses.

2 large zucchini or yellow squash
1 tablespoon extra-virgin olive oil
1 teaspoon minced garlic
¼ cup chopped yellow onion
2 cups chopped tomatoes
½ cup sliced mushrooms
1 cup fresh baby spinach leaves, packed
Salt
Freshly ground black pepper
Pinch crushed red pepper flakes
½ cup crumbled feta cheese
Chopped fresh basil, for garnish

1. Using a vegetable peeler, peel the squash into thin strips; set aside.

2. In a large skillet, heat the oil over medium-high heat.

3. Stir in the garlic and onion, then cook for 6 to 8 minutes until the onion is tender, stirring often.

4. Add the tomatoes, mushrooms, and spinach. Season with salt and pepper and stir in the red pepper flakes. Cook for 2 minutes, or until the spinach is wilted, stirring occasionally.

5. Stir in the cooked squash and cook until just tender, 2 to 3 minutes.

6. Top with feta and basil to serve.

NUTRITION INFO Calories 253, Total Fat 16g, Carbohydrates 21g, Protein 12g, Cholesterol 33mg

Ricotta-Stuffed Spaghetti Squash

SERVES 2   PREP TIME: 15 MINUTES   COOK TIME: 40 MINUTES
MEAL PLAN ● ○ ○

Ricotta is a type of Italian cheese made with whey, the liquid left over after straining curds to make other types of cheese. The process yields a thick, creamy cheese that has a lightly sweet, natural flavor and a high fat content. Ricotta can be made from sheep, cow, goat, or Italian water buffalo milk whey. Because it is so thick and creamy, it makes the perfect filling for these stuffed squash. Blended with fresh spinach and topped with homemade Fresh Tomato Sauce, this recipe makes for a filling meal.

1 large spaghetti squash
1 large egg, lightly beaten
1½ cups ricotta cheese
¼ cup grated Parmesan cheese
1 (10-ounce) package frozen spinach, thawed
2 tablespoons chopped fresh basil
Salt
Freshly ground black pepper
1 cup Fresh Tomato Sauce (page 208)

1. Preheat the oven to 350°F. Cut the spaghetti squash in half lengthwise and scoop out the seeds.

2. Bring a large pot of salted water to a boil. Add the squash halves and boil for 20 minutes, or until the inner flesh is slightly fork tender. Drain and place in a glass dish.

3. While the squash is cooking, prepare the cheese mixture. In a medium mixing bowl, whisk together the egg, ricotta, Parmesan, spinach, and basil.

4. Beat the mixture with an electric hand mixer until light and fluffy. Season with salt and pepper.

5. Spoon the mixture into the cooked squash, and pour the tomato sauce over the top.

6. Bake for 15 to 20 minutes, or until hot and bubbling, and serve.

NUTRITION INFO Calories 517, Total Fat 26g, Carbohydrates 36g, Protein 42g, Cholesterol 171mg

TIP To make the most of this recipe, look for fresh ricotta at your local Italian grocery or specialty foods store. If none of these options is available, you can buy packaged ricotta from your local grocery store. Just be sure it's full-fat and not part-skim ricotta.

Lentil–Brown Rice Casserole

SERVES 2 TO 3   **PREP TIME: 10 MINUTES**   **COOK TIME: 20 MINUTES**
MEAL PLAN ● ○

*This casserole is loaded with vegetarian protein and dietary fiber.
A single ½-cup serving of lentils contains more than 160 percent of
your daily value for molybdenum, 45 percent of your daily value for
folate, and 25 percent of your daily value for phosphorus. Brown rice
is loaded with B vitamins as well as manganese, which plays a role
in energy production in the body and helps promote a healthy
nervous system. In this recipe, you get all of these health benefits
plus the delicious flavors and textures of brown rice and lentils in
one tasty casserole.*

1 (15-ounce) can red lentils, rinsed and drained
1 cup cooked brown rice
½ teaspoon chopped fresh oregano
1 teaspoon minced garlic
Salt
Freshly ground black pepper
¾ cup shredded Cheddar cheese

1. Preheat the oven to 300°F.

2. Combine the lentils, rice, oregano, and garlic in a 9-inch pie
   plate. Season with salt and pepper.

3. Cover the casserole with foil and bake for 10 minutes to
   warm through.

4. Remove the foil and sprinkle the cheese over the casserole.
   Bake for another 10 minutes until the cheese is melted and the
   casserole is hot and bubbling.

5. Let the casserole sit for 5 minutes before serving.

NUTRITION INFO Calories 589, Total Fat 16g, Carbohydrates 79g,
Protein 33g, Cholesterol 45mg

Spiced Chickpeas with Grilled Tofu

SERVES 2   PREP TIME: 5 MINUTES   COOK TIME: 15 MINUTES
MEAL PLAN ● ○

With a punch of vegetarian protein, this dish is sure to keep you full and satisfied. Though the list of ingredients may seem long, this recipe is actually quite simple to make—the long list only means that it's full of flavor. When you first prepare this dish, it's best to serve it warm, but you can serve the leftovers cold just as well. If you're not following the Orange meal plan, feel free to substitute chicken or fish for the grilled tofu in this recipe. To prepare this entire meal indoors, cook the tofu in a cast-iron pan over medium-high heat following the same directions, cooking a few more minutes if needed to heat through.

FOR THE TOFU

2 tablespoons freshly squeezed lemon juice

1 tablespoon extra-virgin olive oil

1 teaspoon minced garlic

Salt

Freshly ground black pepper

8 ounces extra-firm tofu

FOR THE CHICKPEAS

2 tablespoons extra-virgin olive oil

1 medium yellow onion, minced

1 tablespoon minced garlic

1 teaspoon ground coriander

1 teaspoon ground cumin

1 tablespoon freshly squeezed lemon zest

1 (15-ounce) can chickpeas, rinsed and drained

¼ cup vegetable broth

2 cups fresh baby spinach

Lemon wedges, for garnish ▶

To make the tofu

1. Preheat the grill to high heat.

2. In a small bowl, whisk together the lemon juice, oil, and garlic. Season with salt and pepper, and whisk to combine.

3. Slice the tofu into ½-inch pieces and arrange in a glass dish in a single layer.

4. Pour the marinade over the tofu. Cover and chill for 10 minutes.

5. Remove the tofu from the marinade and place the pieces on the grill. Discard the marinade. Cook for 3 to 4 minutes per side until heated through and lightly charred on the edges.

6. Transfer the tofu to a cutting board and coarsely chop.

To make the chickpeas

1. In a large skillet, heat the oil over medium-high heat.

2. Add the onions and garlic and cook for 5 to 6 minutes, stirring often, until the onions begin to soften.

3. Add the coriander, cumin, and lemon zest and cook for 1 minute more, stirring often.

4. Stir in the chickpeas and broth, then cover and simmer for 5 minutes, until heated through.

5. Add the spinach and cook for 2 minutes, or just until the spinach is wilted.

6. Stir in the grilled tofu and serve hot with lemon wedges.

NUTRITION INFO Calories 570, Total Fat 31g, Carbohydrates 47g, Protein 30g, Cholesterol 0mg

Asian Slaw with Thai Tofu

SERVES 2   PREP TIME: 15 MINUTES   COOK TIME: 10 MINUTES
MEAL PLAN ● ●

Tofu is a staple in many Asian cuisines and is known for being an excellent source of vegetarian protein that is very low in fat. As you will see, tofu has a unique consistency and a subtle flavor that absorbs whatever sauce it is cooked in. The Asian Slaw adds a wonderfully cool and crunchy texture to the dish, with just a hint of heat from the crushed red pepper flakes.

FOR THE TOFU

Toasted sesame seeds, for garnish

2 teaspoons extra-virgin olive oil

1 teaspoon sesame oil

½ cup sliced scallions

8 ounces extra-firm tofu, cut into ¾-inch cubes

½ teaspoon crushed red pepper flakes

2 tablespoons almond butter

1 teaspoon grated fresh ginger

2 tablespoons shredded unsweetened coconut

FOR THE SLAW

2 tablespoons rice vinegar

1 teaspoon toasted sesame oil

1 teaspoon grated fresh ginger

Freshly ground black pepper

½ teaspoon crushed red pepper flakes

2 cups shredded napa cabbage

½ cup thinly sliced red bell pepper

¼ cup sliced scallions ▶

To make the tofu

1. In a small skillet, cook the sesame seeds over medium heat for 1 to 2 minutes, stirring often, until lightly browned. Set the seeds aside to cool.

2. In a large skillet, heat the extra-virgin olive oil and the sesame oil over medium-high heat.

3. Reduce the heat to medium, then stir in the scallions and cook for 1 minute.

4. Stir in the tofu and red pepper flakes and cook for 3 to 4 minutes.

5. Whisk in the almond butter and ginger, then remove the skillet from the heat and stir in the shredded coconut.

6. Sprinkle with the toasted sesame seeds.

To make the slaw

1. In a small bowl, whisk together the vinegar, oil, ginger, pepper, and red pepper flakes.

2. Toss the cabbage, bell pepper, and scallions with the dressing in a large salad bowl.

3. Serve with the Thai tofu.

NUTRITION INFO Calories 351, Total Fat 27g, Carbohydrates 13g, Protein 17g, Cholesterol 0mg

Sesame-Ginger Soba Noodles

SERVES 2 **PREP TIME:** 10 **COOK TIME:** 10
MEAL PLAN ● ◔

This Asian-inspired noodle dish is bursting with nutrients and fresh ginger flavor. A touch of creamy almond butter adds a boost of heart-healthy fats. Nutty and tender soba noodles are made from buckwheat flour and, despite the name, they are free of wheat and gluten. Some brands are made with wheat flour, so read labels carefully. If you can't find 100 percent gluten-free, use rice noodles instead.

1 tablespoon almond butter
1 tablespoon wheat-free tamari
Juice of ½ lime
1 teaspoon fresh grated ginger
1 teaspoon sesame oil
1 tablespoon extra-virgin olive oil
6 ounces (dry) soba noodles
½ cup frozen shelled edamame, thawed
¼ cup chopped scallions

1. In a large bowl, make a ginger sauce by whisking together the almond butter, tamari, lime juice, ginger, sesame oil, and olive oil.

2. Cook the soba noodles according to package directions. Drain and add to the bowl with ginger sauce.

3. Add the edamame and scallions and toss well.

4. Serve at room temperature or slightly chilled.

NUTRITION INFO Calories 474, Total Fat 16g, Carbohydrates 70g, Protein 19g, Cholesterol 0mg

Quinoa "Tabbouleh"

SERVES 2   PREP TIME: 15 MINUTES   COOK TIME: 15 MINUTES
MEAL PLAN ● ●

Tabbouleh is a type of Arabic salad traditionally made with bulgur, tomatoes, parsley, and onion. Because wheat products are not allowed on the sugar detox diet, however, this recipe uses quinoa instead of bulgur. Tabbouleh originates from the mountains of Lebanon and Syria, though it has become popular throughout the entire Middle East. There are different variations of the salad around the world, such as meze *in the Arab world, where it is made with romaine lettuce rather than parsley. A Turkish variation on the dish is called* kisir, *and an Armenian variation is known as* eetch.

½ cup uncooked quinoa
1 cup water
¾ cup chopped tomato
¼ cup chopped fresh parsley
½ cup diced English cucumber
2 tablespoons freshly squeezed lemon juice
1 tablespoon sliced scallions
1 tablespoon extra-virgin olive oil
1 teaspoon minced yellow onion
Salt
Freshly ground black pepper

1. In a small saucepan, stir together the quinoa and water. Bring to a boil, then reduce the heat to low and cover for 15 minutes.

2. Turn off the heat and let the quinoa sit for 5 minutes, until it has absorbed all of the water.

3. Fluff the quinoa with a fork and allow to cool.

4. In a large mixing bowl, combine the tomato, parsley, cucumber, lemon juice, scallions, oil, and onion. Season with salt and pepper, and toss with the cooked quinoa.

5. Serve warm or chill until ready to serve.

NUTRITION INFO Calories 229, Total Fat 10g, Carbohydrates 30g, Protein 7g, Cholesterol 0mg

TIP If you don't have any English cucumbers on hand, you can simply remove the seeds from a regular cucumber. To do so, cut the cucumber into lengthwise quarters, then trim the middle ½ inch or so of each quarter to remove the seeds.

Ratatouille

SERVES 2   PREP TIME: 20 MINUTES   COOK TIME: 50 MINUTES
MEAL PLAN ● ◐ ◌

Ratatouille is a traditional French dish originating in Nice—the full name of the dish is actually ratatouille Niçoise. Traditionally made from stewed vegetables, ratatouille works equally well as a main dish or a side dish. The key to making it authentic is to cook each of the vegetables separately to ensure they retain their individual flavor. If you're in a hurry, you can cook the veggies together, but the overall flavor of the dish won't be quite the same. To make the recipe dairy-free, and Blue-plan friendly, skip the feta and garnish with chopped cashews.

FOR THE SAUCE

1½ pounds ripe tomatoes
1 tablespoon extra-virgin olive oil
1 garlic clove, minced
½ cup chopped fresh parsley
½ cup fresh basil leaves, torn in half

FOR THE RATATOUILLE

1 large eggplant, cut into 1-inch cubes
1 teaspoon coarse salt
1 tablespoon extra-virgin olive oil
1 medium yellow onion, sliced thin
2 assorted bell peppers, cut into 1-inch chunks
1 large yellow squash, cut into 1-inch chunks
2 cups fresh baby spinach
¼ cup crumbled feta cheese

To make the sauce

1. Use a sharp knife to cut an "X" into the top of each tomato.

2. In a large pot of boiling water, blanch the tomatoes for 1 minute. Using a slotted spoon, move the tomatoes to a plate and allow to cool.

3. Peel the skins from the tomatoes, then coarsely chop them.

4. In a large skillet, heat the oil over medium heat.

5. Stir in the garlic, parsley, basil, and blanched tomatoes and cook for 10 minutes, stirring occasionally, until thickened.

To make the ratatouille

1. Toss the eggplant with the salt in a large colander and let stand for 10 minutes.

2. In a large skillet, heat the oil over medium heat, then stir in the onions and cook for 10 minutes until softened.

3. Add the bell peppers and yellow squash to the skillet and cook for 10 minutes, stirring often.

4. Pat the eggplant dry with a paper towel, then add the eggplant to the skillet and cook for 10 minutes until softened, stirring occasionally.

5. Stir in the tomato sauce and fresh spinach and simmer over low heat, covered, for 10 minutes, until the vegetables are very tender.

6. Top the ratatouille with the crumbled feta.

NUTRITION INFO Calories 374, Total Fat 20g, Carbohydrates 48g, Protein 13g, Cholesterol 17mg

Ratatouille-Stuffed Peppers

SERVES 2   PREP TIME: 15 MINUTES   COOK TIME: 30 MINUTES
MEAL PLAN ● ●

This recipe is the perfect way to use leftovers from the Ratatouille recipe in this book. Many recipes for stuffed peppers utilize plain tomato sauce for moisture and flavor, but this recipe is enhanced by the ratatouille, which is made from a variety of vegetables, not just tomatoes. Once you try this dish, you may find that you don't have the desire to eat "regular" stuffed peppers again.

> 4 assorted bell peppers
> 1 cup Ratatouille (see page 144)
> 1 cup cooked brown rice
> ½ cup shredded mozzarella cheese

1. Preheat the oven to 350°F.

2. Slice the tops off the peppers and carefully remove the cores and seeds. Arrange the peppers upright in a large glass baking dish.

3. In a medium mixing bowl, stir together the ratatouille and brown rice.

4. Spoon the rice mixture into the peppers and sprinkle with the mozzarella cheese.

5. Fill the baking dish with about a quarter inch of water, then bake for 30 minutes or until the filling is hot.

NUTRITION INFO Calories 406, Total Fat 13g, Carbohydrates 58g, Protein 15g, Cholesterol 15mg

TIP Don't add too much water to the baking dish, or your peppers may become mushy as they cook. The water will effectively steam the peppers while they are in the oven, and if you add too much water, it won't evaporate properly during the allotted cooking time.

Tempeh and Swiss Chard Stir-Fry

SERVES 2   PREP TIME: 5 MINUTES   COOK TIME: 15 MINUTES
MEAL PLAN   ● ○ ○ ●

Tempeh is a delicious soy-based protein option for those who might want a break from tofu. It has a heartier texture and nuttier flavor and is more versatile than you might think. Pair it up with a superfood like Swiss chard, and you'll have a stir-fry that is so satisfying, you won't need to have rice along with it.

1 tablespoon olive oil

1 garlic clove, minced

1-inch piece ginger root, minced

8 ounces tempeh, diced

½ yellow onion, sliced

1 large bunch of Swiss chard (leaves and stems), chopped

1 teaspoon sesame oil

2 tablespoons coconut aminos

Juice of ½ a lime

2 teaspoons sesame seeds

1. In a large pan or wok, heat the oil, add the garlic and ginger, and sauté for 30 seconds.

2. Add the tempeh, and cook for 2 minutes more.

3. Add the onion and Swiss chard, and continue to cook to slightly wilt the greens.

4. Add the sesame oil, coconut aminos, and lime juice.

5. Toss and allow to cook for 6 to 8 minutes, until the ingredients are warmed through.

6. Add the sesame seeds, toss, and serve.

NUTRITION INFO Calories 362, Total Fat 23g, Carbohydrates 20g, Protein 26g, Cholesterol 0mg

Spinach and White Bean Stew

SERVES 2   PREP TIME: 10 MINUTES   COOK TIME: 30 MINUTES
MEAL PLAN ● ●

White cannellini beans are related to the kidney bean and are particularly popular in southern Italy. These beans are the most abundant plant-based source of phosphatidylserine, a phospholipid component that may provide significant benefits for memory and cognition. In addition to containing a variety of nutrients, these beans are high in protein but low in fat, which makes them a great ingredient to use if you're trying to lose weight on the sugar detox. If you prefer to use dried beans, soak overnight, add 2 cups of water, and increase cooking time by one hour.

2 tablespoons extra-virgin olive oil

½ medium yellow onion, grated

1 garlic clove, minced

1 medium ripe tomato, diced

1 tablespoon chopped fresh parsley

1 tablespoon chopped fresh cilantro

1 teaspoon coarse salt

1 teaspoon paprika

1 teaspoon ground cumin

½ teaspoon ground ginger

Pinch cayenne pepper

1 (15-ounce) can no-salt-added cannellini beans, rinsed and drained

2 cups fresh baby spinach leaves, packed

¼ cup crumbled feta cheese

1. In a large skillet, heat the oil over medium heat.

2. Stir in the onion and garlic and cook for 5 minutes, then add the tomatoes, parsley, cilantro, and salt, paprika, cumin, ginger, and cayenne pepper.

3. Add the beans, then bring the mixture to a boil.

4. Reduce the heat and simmer for 30 minutes, then stir in the fresh spinach.

5. Spoon into bowls and top with the crumbled feta to serve.

NUTRITION INFO Calories 381, Total Fat 19g, Carbohydrates 40g, Protein 17g, Cholesterol 17mg

Quinoa Cakes

These tender quinoa cakes are elegant enough for company but easy enough to throw together for a weeknight meal. Sweet potatoes add a hint of natural sweetness while helping the cakes hold together. The sweet potatoes are packed with nutrients, including vitamins A and C and potassium, and with its high fiber and balance of amino acids, it's no wonder the United Nations declared 2013 the International Year of Quinoa!

3 teaspoons extra-virgin olive oil, divided
½ yellow onion, finely chopped
Coarse salt
2 cups cooked quinoa
½ cup shredded sweet potato
½ teaspoon paprika
1 large egg
¼ teaspoon freshly ground black pepper
Mixed greens, for serving

1. Heat 1 teaspoon of oil in a nonstick skillet.

2. Add the onion, season with salt, and sauté until translucent, about 3 minutes; set aside to cool.

3. Combine the cooked onion, quinoa, sweet potato, paprika, and egg in a food processor fitted with a steel blade.

4. Season with the salt and black pepper.

5. Pulse until the mixture is well combined.

6. Form the mixture into 6 equal-sized patties (about ½ cup each).

7. Heat 2 teaspoons of oil in a large skillet. Place 2 cakes in the skillet and cook for 5 minutes per side. Transfer to a plate.

8. Repeat for the remaining cakes, and serve over a bed of mixed greens.

NUTRITION INFO Calories 453, Total Fat 15g, Carbohydrates 66g, Protein 16g, Cholesterol 93mg

White Chili

SERVES 2 PREP TIME: 10 MINUTES COOK TIME: 30 MINUTES
MEAL PLAN ● ○

Yes, there is such thing as a tomato-less chili. You can find tomatillos in the produce section of most large chain grocery stores, and their tangy, fresh flavor is second to none. This chili is vegetarian but pleasantly hearty, perfect for a cool evening meal. For even better texture, puree half of the beans and leave the rest whole. The pureed mixture will further thicken the chili.

1 tablespoon extra-virgin olive oil
1 yellow onion, diced
2 medium stalks celery, chopped
1 poblano pepper, diced
3 tomatillos, husks removed and diced
2 garlic cloves, minced
1 teaspoon ground cumin
¼ teaspoon cayenne pepper
Coarse salt
3 cups vegetable or chicken broth
1 (15-ounce) can cannellini beans, rinsed and drained
1 (15-ounce) can pinto beans, rinsed and drained
¼ cup chopped cilantro

1. In a stockpot over medium heat, heat the oil. Add the onion, celery, pepper, tomatillos, and garlic.

2. Season with salt and pepper and cook for 2 minutes.

3. Add the cumin and cayenne, season with salt, and cook for an additional 3 to 4 minutes.

4. Add the broth, cannellini beans, and pinto beans, and stir well to combine.

5. Bring to a simmer, reduce heat, and cook for 20 to 25 minutes.

6. Add the cilantro just before serving.

NUTRITION INFO Calories 510, Total Fat 11g, Carbohydrates 71g, Protein 30g, Cholesterol 0mg

TEN

SEAFOOD & FISH

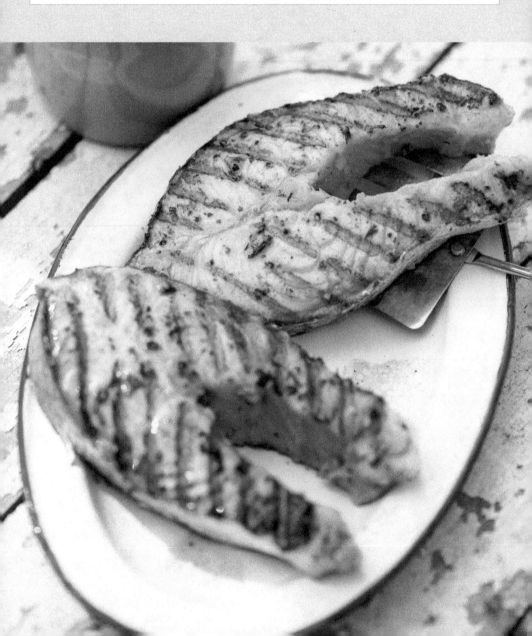

Shrimp Scampi 156

Baked White Fish Fillets 158

Chile-Lime Grilled Salmon 160

Herb-Marinated Cod 162

Simple Roasted Salmon with Tomatoes 163

Blackened Salmon with Cucumber Salsa 164

Grilled Shrimp with Olives and Feta 166

Steamed Mussels with Saffron 167

Cod and Green Beans in Parchment 168

Spinach Salad with Shrimp 170

Spicy Salmon Burgers 171

Shrimp Scampi

SERVES 2   PREP TIME: 5 MINUTES   COOK TIME: 10 MINUTES
MEAL PLAN ● ◐

Shrimp scampi is a dish that sounds Italian but is actually more Italian-American. The name of the dish is derived from the type of seafood that was originally used to prepare the dish—scampi, also known as langoustines. Though original 1970s versions of the dish consisted of little more than shrimp, olive oil, and garlic, modern shrimp scampi is often bathed in butter. In this recipe, however, you will find the dish is closer to the original—cooked in coconut oil rather than butter, and seasoned with garlic and freshly ground black pepper.

2 tablespoons coconut oil

1 teaspoon minced garlic

12 ounces uncooked shrimp, peeled and deveined

¼ cup low-sodium chicken or vegetable broth

¼ teaspoon coarse salt

¼ teaspoon freshly ground black pepper

⅓ cup grated Parmesan cheese

1 tablespoon fresh chopped parsley

1. In a large skillet, melt the oil over medium heat.

2. Add the garlic and cook for 1 minute, until fragrant.

3. Place the shrimp in the skillet and cook for 1 minute, then turn the shrimp over and cook for another 1 to 2 minutes until evenly pink.

4. Increase the heat to high and add the broth.

5. Season the shrimp with salt and pepper and simmer for 30 to 60 seconds until most of the broth has cooked off.

6. Remove the skillet from the heat, and stir in the cheese and parsley before serving.

NUTRITION INFO Calories 419, Total Fat 23g, Carbohydrates 5g, Protein 49g, Cholesterol 378mg

TIP If you're no longer detoxing and want to make this recipe, you can substitute 1 cup of dry white wine for the broth and cook according to the directions. The wine will naturally add some sweetness to the dish. It will cook off more than the broth, so that's why the recipe calls for a higher quantity.

Baked White Fish Fillets

SERVES 2   PREP TIME: 10 MINUTES   COOK TIME: 20 MINUTES
MEAL PLAN ● ●

If you're trying to lose weight while on the sugar detox, fish is going to be your best friend. In addition to being tender and full of flavor, fish is rich in protein. It's incredibly easy to prepare, and in most recipes the types of fish are interchangeable. In this recipe, for example, you might use tilapia or haddock, but you could just as easily substitute any other type of white fish, such as halibut or cod. Having so many options ensures that you don't have to eat the same meal week after week.

> 2 (6-ounce) boneless white fish fillets
>   (such as tilapia or haddock)
> ¼ cup sour cream
> 2 tablespoons coconut oil
> 10 ounces fresh baby spinach, chopped
> ½ teaspoon paprika
> Salt
> Freshly ground black pepper
> Juice of ½ lemon

1. Preheat the oven to 350°F.

2. Dip the fish fillets in sour cream until coated and allow to rest for 30 minutes.

3. In a large skillet, melt the oil over medium-high heat. Add the spinach and cook for 2 minutes, until wilted.

4. Spread the wilted spinach in the bottom of a 9-by-13-inch baking dish and arrange the fillets on top.

5. Add the paprika to the skillet with the oil, season with salt and pepper, and cook for 30 seconds.

6. Drizzle the hot oil over the fish and spritz with the lemon juice.

7. Bake for 20 minutes, or until the fish is cooked through. Serve hot.

NUTRITION INFO Calories 349, Total Fat 20g, Carbohydrates 7g, Protein 36g, Cholesterol 13mg

TIP It's best to avoid high-fat products like sour cream if you're trying to lose weight. In this recipe, you may substitute plain Greek yogurt for the sour cream and follow the same instructions.

Chile-Lime Grilled Salmon

SERVES 2   PREP TIME: 5 MINUTES   COOK TIME: 15 MINUTES
MEAL PLAN ● ● ●

If you believe that fish is difficult to prepare, this recipe for Chile-Lime Grilled Salmon will convince you that this simply isn't true! With just 5 minutes of preparation and 15 minutes of cooking time, you can create a healthy, flavorful meal that will help you fill your protein quota for the day without overloading you with calories. This grilled salmon is lightly flavored with chili powder and cumin as well as garlic and fresh lime juice—you don't want anything too heavy that will overpower the natural flavor of the fish.

Extra-virgin olive oil, for seasoning
2 (6-ounce) boneless salmon fillets
2 tablespoons freshly squeezed lime juice
1 garlic clove, minced
½ teaspoon chili powder
½ teaspoon ground cumin
½ teaspoon coarse salt
½ teaspoon freshly ground black pepper
Fresh lime wedges, for garnish

1. Preheat your grill to high heat and season the grates with olive oil.

2. Rinse the fillets, then pat dry with paper towels.

3. In a small bowl, whisk together the lime juice, garlic, chili powder, cumin, salt, and pepper and brush liberally over the fillets.

4. Grill the fillets for 5 to 7 minutes on each side, until the flesh flakes easily with a fork.

5. Serve the fish with fresh lime wedges.

    NUTRITION INFO Calories 253, Total Fat 13g, Carbohydrates 1g, Protein 33g, Cholesterol 75mg

TIP If you don't have a grill, you can easily make a baked version of this dish. Preheat your oven to 350°F. Place the fillets in a glass baking dish, and pour the lime juice, garlic, and spices over them. Bake for 12 to 15 minutes, until the flesh flakes easily with a fork. Serve hot with fresh lime wedges.

Herb-Marinated Cod

SERVES 2   PREP TIME: 20 MINUTES   COOK TIME: 15 MINUTES
MEAL PLAN ● ● ●

This is the most unintimidating fish recipe that you'll ever come across. The mild flavor of cod pairs well with herbs and citrus, and it cooks up easily whether it's grilled, broiled, roasted, or steamed. Cut into 4 pieces or cook whole. Add thinly sliced vegetables, and they will cook along with the fish. For an especially easy cleanup, wrap the fish in foil packets and toss them on the grill.

2 tablespoons extra-virgin olive oil
Juice of ½ lemon
1 teaspoon ground fennel
1 tablespoon chopped fresh tarragon
Salt
Freshly ground black pepper
12 ounces fresh cod

1. In a large bowl, combine the olive oil, lemon juice, fennel, and tarragon. Season with salt and pepper and whisk well.

2. Place the fish in a large plastic bag along with the marinade.

3. Marinate in the refrigerator for at least 15 minutes, or up to 1 hour.

4. Grill or broil for 5 to 7 minutes per side, until just cooked through.

NUTRITION INFO Calories 305, Total Fat 16g, Carbohydrates 1g, Protein 39g, Cholesterol 94mg

Simple Roasted Salmon with Tomatoes

SERVES 2   PREP TIME: 5 MINUTES   COOK TIME: 20 MINUTES
MEAL PLAN ⊙ ⊙ ●

Preparing salmon does not have to be difficult or stressful. Ask the fish-monger to remove the skin, and you can go from the fridge to the oven in minutes. Use this method with any combo of veggies and fresh herbs. Green beans and tarragon are another fabulous combination.

2 (6-ounce) boneless salmon fillets, skin removed

3 teaspoons extra-virgin olive oil, divided

Coarse salt

Freshly ground black pepper

1 pint cherry tomatoes, halved

1 garlic clove, minced

½ cup fresh basil leaves, torn

1. Preheat the oven to 400°F.

2. Lay the salmon fillets in a baking dish and drizzle each with 1 teaspoon of oil, then season with salt and pepper.

3. In a small bowl, combine the cherry tomatoes, garlic, and the remaining 1 teaspoon of oil and season with salt and pepper. Toss well to coat.

4. Pour the tomatoes over the salmon and roast for 20 minutes, or until the salmon is cooked as desired.

5. Remove from the oven, top with fresh basil, and serve.

NUTRITION INFO Calories 315, Total Fat 18g, Carbohydrates 7g, Protein 35g, Cholesterol 75mg

Blackened Salmon with Cucumber Salsa

SERVES 2   PREP TIME: 10 MINUTES   COOK TIME: 15 MINUTES
MEAL PLAN ○ ○ ●

There is something magical about the combination of salmon and cucumber. Cool, crisp cukes take on an even more important role by helping put out the flames from a spicy dry rub. Scale up the recipe for the dry spice mix. It's delicious on chicken and veggies as well, so you will want to keep some on hand.

FOR THE SALSA

1 large cucumber, finely diced

2 tablespoons finely chopped onion

2 tablespoons chopped cilantro

2 teaspoons rice vinegar

Coarse salt

Freshly ground black pepper

FOR THE SALMON

1 teaspoon ground fennel

1 teaspoon ground ginger

½ teaspoon onion powder

½ teaspoon mustard powder

½ teaspoon coarse salt

½ teaspoon freshly ground black pepper

2 (6-ounce) boneless salmon fillets, skin removed

To make the salsa

1. In a small bowl, stir together the cucumber, onion, cilantro, and vinegar.

2. Season with salt and pepper and set aside.

To make the salmon

1. In a small bowl, mix together the fennel, ginger, onion powder, mustard powder, salt, and pepper.

2. Preheat the grill or grill pan to medium-high.

3. Gently rub the spice mixture on the salmon so that it evenly coats each side.

4. Grill for 4 minutes, then turn and cook on the other side for an additional 4 minutes.

5. Serve topped with salsa.

NUTRITION INFO Calories 269, Total Fat 11g, Carbohydrates 9g, Protein 35g, Cholesterol 75mg

TIP Dry spice rubs are a great way to impart a lot of flavor when you don't have the time to marinate a piece of fish. A quick sprinkle of some bold flavors goes a long way!

Grilled Shrimp with Olives and Feta

SERVES 2 PREP TIME: 10 MINUTES COOK TIME: 10 MINUTES
MEAL PLAN ◦ ●

Shrimp are healthy kitchen all-stars! They are high in protein and low in fat, and they cook up in minutes. Grilling them at a high heat brings out their natural sweetness, which is then perfectly balanced out by the savory olives and some pleasantly pungent feta cheese.

12 ounces large shrimp, peeled and deveined
2 tablespoons extra-virgin olive oil, divided
Coarse salt
Freshly ground black pepper
1 (4-ounce) piece feta cheese, diced
1 cup kalamata olives
2 cups arugula
1 tablespoon chopped fresh oregano
2 teaspoons vinegar (red wine or balsamic suggested)

1. Heat the grill or grill pan to high heat.

2. Drizzle the shrimp with 1 tablespoon of olive oil and season with salt and pepper.

3. Grill the shrimp for 2 to 3 minutes per side, or until opaque, and set aside to cool slightly.

4. In a large bowl, combine the feta, olives, arugula, remaining 1 tablespoon of olive oil, oregano, and vinegar. Toss well and serve with the shrimp.

NUTRITION INFO Calories 497, Total Fat 34g, Carbohydrates 12g, Protein 41g, Cholesterol 293mg

Steamed Mussels with Saffron

SERVES 2   PREP TIME: 10 MINUTES   COOK TIME: 15 MINUTES
MEAL PLAN ○ ○ ●

If you love shellfish, this is the recipe for you. Purveyed from flowers, saffron is a one-of-a-kind spice with tremendous flavor. Serve these tender steamed mussels alone for a light meal or along with a bowl of soup or salad for something more substantial.

1 pound mussels, scrubbed clean

¾ teaspoon coarse salt

1 fennel bulb, thinly sliced

2 garlic cloves, chopped

5 sprigs fresh thyme

2 teaspoons saffron

2 cups fish or chicken stock

1. Place the mussels in the bottom of a large soup pot.

2. Add the salt, fennel, garlic, thyme, and saffron to the pot and stir gently.

3. Pour in the stock, and turn the heat on to high.

4. Once the mixture begins to boil, reduce the heat to medium, cover, and allow to steam for 10 to 12 minutes, or until the mussels are open. Discard any mussels that do not open after 10 to 15 minutes of cooking.

5. Serve warm.

NUTRITION INFO Calories 248, Total Fat 6g, Carbohydrates 19g, Protein 29g, Cholesterol 64mg

Cod and Green Beans in Parchment

SERVES 2   PREP TIME: 10 MINUTES   COOK TIME: 20 MINUTES
MEAL PLAN ● ● ●

Steaming food in packets of parchment is easy, mess-free, and one of the healthiest cooking methods around. Don't be intimidated by cooking in parchment. Try it once, and you'll be hooked. The best part is, it saves on clean-up time as well. Go from the oven to the plate, and allow diners to open up their own little present.

2 (6-ounce) cod fillets
2 cups green beans, trimmed and chopped
2 sprigs fresh thyme
2 tablespoons extra-virgin olive oil, divided
Coarse salt
Freshly ground black pepper

1. Preheat the oven to 400°F.

2. Fold two rectangular pieces of parchment paper in half to create a crease down the middle.

3. To make a packet, place the fish on one side of the parchment paper and scatter the green beans on top.

4. Top with a sprig of fresh thyme.

5. Drizzle with 1 tablespoon of oil and season generously with salt and pepper.

6. Fold the parchment over the fish, then gently fold over the edges to close, creating a half-moon-shaped packet.

7. Repeat with the remaining piece of fish.

8. Place both packets on a baking sheet and bake for 20 minutes.

9. Allow to rest for 5 minutes before serving.

NUTRITION INFO Calories 321, Total Fat 16g, Carbohydrates 8g, Protein 39g, Cholesterol 0mg

Spinach Salad with Shrimp

SERVES I   PREP TIME: 10 MINUTES
MEAL PLAN ⬤

Next time you prepare shrimp, make a double batch so you have leftovers for this salad. Instead of green olives, try Lemon-Marinated Olives (page 98) for an extra kick. When making a salad, don't leave out the salad greens when you season or dress the rest of your ingredients. Seasoning the greens, too, will make a huge difference in the flavor of the entire recipe.

1 tablespoon extra-virgin olive oil

Juice of ½ lemon

Coarse salt

Freshly ground black pepper

3 cups baby spinach

½ cup canned chickpeas, rinsed and drained

¼ cup green olives

4 ounces cooked shrimp

1. Place the olive oil and lemon juice in a medium bowl.

2. Season with salt and pepper and whisk well to combine.

3. Add the spinach and toss well to coat in the dressing.

4. Add the chickpeas, olives, and shrimp, season with salt and pepper again, and toss well.

NUTRITION INFO Calories 416, Total Fat 22g, Carbohydrates 22g, Protein 35g, Cholesterol 239mg

Spicy Salmon Burgers

SERVES 2   PREP TIME: 10 MINUTES   COOK TIME: 15 MINUTES
MEAL PLAN   ● ● ●

In under 30 minutes, you can prep and serve up these healthy burgers with a kick of heat. Even after your detox, you're likely to come back to these satisfying crispy patties in crunchy lettuce wraps again and again.

8 ounces raw salmon, skin removed, diced
1 tablespoon freshly squeezed lemon juice
1 large egg
1 slice grain-free, gluten-free bread, torn
½ jalapeño pepper, finely chopped
¼ cup chopped onion
½ teaspoon coarse salt
½ teaspoon black pepper
1 tablespoon coconut oil
Lettuce leaves, for wrapping
Lemon wedges, for garnish

1. Using a food processor, pulse the salmon, lemon juice, egg, bread, jalapeño pepper, onion, salt, and pepper until well combined.

2. Transfer the mixture to a bowl and form into two patties.

3. Heat the coconut oil in a skillet over medium heat.

4. Cook the burgers for 7 to 8 minutes per side.

5. Serve wrapped in lettuce leaves and garnished with fresh lemon.

NUTRITION INFO Calories 293, Total Fat 17g, Carbohydrates 9g, Protein 26g, Cholesterol 143mg

ELEVEN

POULTRY & MEAT

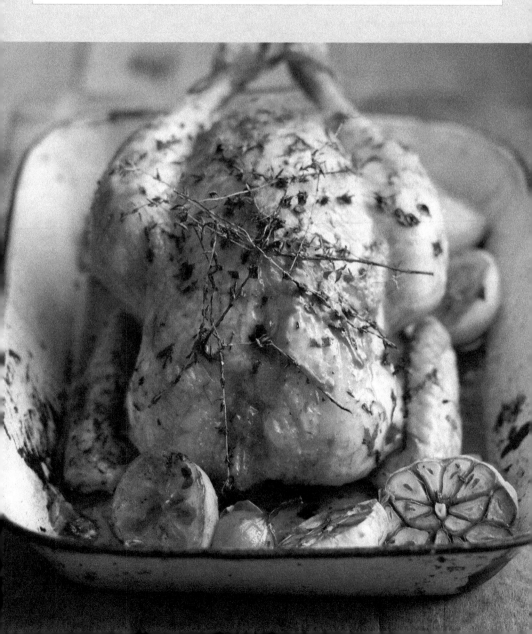

Lemon-Thyme Roasted Chicken *174*

Chicken Fajita Lettuce Cups *175*

Hobo Packets *176*

Creamy Spinach and Bacon Pie *177*

Curry-Ginger Pork Chops *178*

Grilled Garlic-Rosemary Pork Tenderloin
with Steamed Broccoli *179*

Argentinean-Style Beef *181*

Meatballs, Your Way *182*

Ground Beef Casserole with Cheese Crust *183*

Turkey Meatloaf *184*

Asian Chicken Kebabs *185*

Slow-Cooker Pot Roast *186*

Chicken Sausage Patties *187*

Pesto Grilled Chicken Thighs *188*

Lemon-Thyme Roasted Chicken

SERVES 4   PREP TIME: 10 MINUTES   COOK TIME: 1 HOUR 30 MINUTES
MEAL PLAN ● ● ●

If you've never roasted a whole chicken before, this recipe is the perfect place to start. The preparation method is quick and uncomplicated—just what you need as a beginner. If you're only cooking for yourself, don't think that rules out this recipe. Enjoy the chicken while it's hot, and save the leftovers for use in other recipes, like Chicken Salad with Walnuts (page 109) or even homemade chicken soup. Once you try it, you may find yourself cooking a roasted chicken almost every week simply because it's so easy, there's no reason not to!

1 (5- to 6-pound) roasting chicken
Salt
Freshly ground black pepper
2 lemons
4 sprigs fresh thyme
2 to 3 tablespoons coconut oil

1. Preheat the oven to 425°F.

2. Remove the giblets from the chicken cavity and rinse the bird in cool water, inside and out. Pat dry with clean paper towels.

3. Season the chicken inside and out with salt and pepper, then cut the lemons in half and place them inside the cavity with the thyme.

4. Close the cavity with string, and rub the oil all over the chicken.

5. Cook for 1 hour and 30 minutes, until the juices run clear.

6. Let the chicken rest for 10 minutes on a cutting board before carving and serving.

NUTRITION INFO Calories 749, Total Fat 64g, Carbohydrates 0g, Protein 81g, Cholesterol 385mg

Chicken Fajita Lettuce Cups

SERVES 2 PREP TIME: 10 MINUTES COOK TIME: 15 MINUTES
MEAL PLAN ◔ ◔ ●

This recipe offers a refreshing spin on a classic. Keep these fajitas light and crunchy by skipping the highly processed flour tortillas. Wrap the high-protein, low-fat chicken in crisp lettuce leaves for a satisfying, guilt-free meal.

1 tablespoon coconut oil

2 large boneless, skinless chicken breasts, sliced

2 tablespoons coconut aminos

1 tablespoon rice vinegar

Pinch red pepper flakes

2 large bell peppers, sliced

½ red onion, sliced

1 head green leaf lettuce (leaves separated), for serving

1. In a large skillet over medium-high heat, heat the oil.

2. Add the sliced chicken and cook until browned on all sides, about 4 to 5 minutes.

3. Season with the coconut aminos, vinegar, and red pepper and continue to cook for an additional 5 minutes.

4. Add the peppers and onion and sauté until the chicken is cooked through and the vegetables are slightly tender, about 5 minutes more.

5. Serve wrapped in the lettuce leaves.

NUTRITION INFO Calories 590, Total Fat 24g, Carbohydrates 18g, Protein 70g, Cholesterol 202mg

Hobo Packets

SERVES 2   PREP TIME: 5 MINUTES   COOK TIME: 20 MINUTES
MEAL PLAN ◌ ◌ ●

If you aren't much of a cook, you will love this recipe because it requires virtually no cooking skill. A hobo packet is simply a packet of foil containing meat, vegetables, and seasoning cooked in the oven. This recipe can be adapted for other kinds of poultry, including turkey; you can even use it for fish, though you'll need to reduce the baking time to avoid overcooking. Feel free to season the chicken as you like with chili powder or a pinch of cayenne pepper to give it a little kick.

2 boneless skinless chicken breasts
1 tablespoon coconut oil, divided
Salt
Freshly ground black pepper
Chili powder or cayenne pepper, for seasoning (optional)
2 cups mixed chopped vegetables

1. Preheat the oven to 375°F.

2. Cut two large pieces of aluminum foil and place a chicken breast in the center of each.

3. Top each chicken breast with ½ tablespoon of oil and season with salt and pepper. Season with the chili powder or cayenne pepper (if using).

4. Spoon 1 cup of vegetables on top of each chicken breast, then fold the foil into a packet around the chicken.

5. Bake the packets on a baking sheet for 18 to 20 minutes, until the chicken is cooked through.

6. Let cool slightly and serve.

NUTRITION INFO Calories 446, Total Fat 18g, Carbohydrates 24g, Protein 46g, Cholesterol 126mg

Creamy Spinach and Bacon Pie

SERVES 2   PREP TIME: 5 MINUTES   COOK TIME: 30 MINUTES
MEAL PLAN ● ●

Once your detox is over, this is a great recipe to double, even if you're just cooking for yourself. This is because it's so easy to reheat. Simply store the leftovers in an airtight container in the refrigerator and reheat one slice at a time, as needed. Using this method, you can enjoy a hot dinner and several tasty lunches from only a single recipe. What could be simpler than that?

4 slices uncooked bacon, chopped
2 tablespoons chopped yellow onion
1 cup chopped baby spinach
¼ cup whole milk
6 large eggs, lightly beaten
Salt
Freshly ground black pepper
½ cup grated Cheddar cheese

1. Preheat the oven to 400°F.

2. In a large ovenproof skillet, heat the bacon over medium-high heat and cook until crisp. Remove the bacon with a slotted spoon.

3. Stir in the onion and cook for 5 minutes until tender, then stir in the spinach and cook for another 2 minutes until it has wilted.

4. In a small bowl, whisk together the milk, eggs, salt, and pepper.

5. Add the egg mixture to the pan and gently scramble for 2 to 3 minutes.

6. Sprinkle with the Cheddar cheese and bacon.

7. Bake for 10 to 15 minutes until the cheese is melted and the eggs are set.

NUTRITION INFO Calories 406, Total Fat 29g, Carbohydrates 5g, Protein 31g, Cholesterol 601mg

Curry-Ginger Pork Chops

SERVES 2   PREP TIME: 20 MINUTES   COOK TIME: 15 MINUTES
MEAL PLAN ● ● ●

If you're tired of meals based around chicken and beef, why not give pork a try? Pork is an excellent source of protein and contains a variety of nutrients. A 3-ounce serving of pork contains only 4 grams of fat but more than 40 percent of your daily value for protein. Pork is also a great source of B vitamins, which help create red blood cells and play an important role in the metabolism of food in the body. If the health benefits of pork aren't enough to convince you, then the flavor of these Curry-Ginger Pork Chops will!

2 tablespoons coconut oil, divided
2 (6-ounce) boneless pork chops
1 medium yellow onion, sliced thin
2 tablespoons fresh minced ginger
1 teaspoon curry powder
⅓ cup low-sodium chicken broth

1. In a large skillet, heat 1 tablespoon oil over medium-high heat.

2. Add the pork chops and cook for 2 minutes on each side to sear; transfer the seared chops to a plate.

3. Reduce the skillet temperature to medium and stir in the remaining 1 tablespoon oil along with the onions, ginger, and curry powder.

4. Cook for 10 minutes, stirring often, until the onions are tender.

5. Return the chops to the skillet and pour in the broth.

6. Cover and simmer over low heat for 15 minutes, or until the pork is cooked through, and serve.

NUTRITION INFO Calories 409, Total Fat 20g, Carbohydrates 10g, Protein 46g, Cholesterol 124mg

Grilled Garlic-Rosemary Pork Tenderloin with Steamed Broccoli

SERVES 2 TO 3   **PREP TIME: 10 MINUTES**   **COOK TIME: 20 MINUTES**
MEAL PLAN ● ● ●

Consider this recipe yet another example of why detoxing does not mean you can't enjoy a truly hearty meal. The high heat of the grill will seal in the juices, keeping this lean cut of pork tender and full of flavor. The combination of rosemary and garlic provides a potent blend of cell-protecting antioxidants.

Salt
Freshly ground black pepper
2 tablespoons coconut oil
1 tablespoon chopped garlic
1 tablespoon chopped fresh rosemary
1 pork tenderloin (about 1 pound)
3 cups broccoli florets

1. Preheat the grill or grill pan over medium-high heat.

2. Season generously with salt and pepper.

3. In a small saucepan, heat the coconut oil, garlic, and rosemary.

4. With a brush, slather the pork tenderloin with the garlic and herb mixture.

5. Transfer to the grill and cook for 4 to 5 minutes per side, until the internal temperature reaches 145°F.

6. Allow the pork to rest for 10 minutes before slicing.

7. While the pork rests, fill a medium saucepan with about 1 inch of water and bring to a simmer. ▶

8. Put the broccoli florets in a steamer basket, cover, and cook until tender, about 10 to 12 minutes.

9. Remove the broccoli from the steamer basket and season with salt and pepper, if desired.

10. Serve the pork and broccoli together.

    NUTRITION INFO Calories 500, Total Fat 22g, Carbohydrates 12g, Protein 64g, Cholesterol 166mg

Argentinean-Style Beef

SERVES 2 PREP TIME: 30 MINUTES COOK TIME: 10 MINUTES
MEAL PLAN ○ ○ ●

Argentina is currently the third largest exporter of beef in the world, and the cattle industry plays a key role in the country's economy and culture. Argentine beef is traditionally cooked over an open flame, as in this recipe, and is often served with a chimichurri sauce like the one you will find on page 213.

1 pound flank steak
2 lemons, halved
Coarse salt

1. Rinse the steaks and pat dry, then squeeze the lemon juice over them and sprinkle with salt.

2. Let the steaks sit at room temperature for 30 minutes.

3. Preheat the grill or grill pan to high heat and place the steaks on the hot grates.

4. Cook for 2 to 3 minutes on each side, then let the steaks rest for 5 minutes or so on a cutting board to continue cooking to medium-rare.

5. Slice the meat against the grain to serve.

NUTRITION INFO Calories 457, Total Fat 19g, Carbohydrates 5g, Protein 64g, Cholesterol 125mg

TIP For other cuts, such as flat-iron, T-bone, or skirt steaks, sear the steaks for 1 to 2 minutes on each side, then move the steaks away from direct heat and cook for another 2 minutes for medium-rare. Let the steaks rest for 5 minutes before slicing.

Meatballs, Your Way

MAKES 12 MEATBALLS (2–3 PER SERVING)
PREP TIME: 10 MINUTES   COOK TIME: 15 MINUTES
MEAL PLAN ● ●

Meatballs are a staple item that everyone should know how to prepare because they are so versatile. Enjoy your meatballs on their own with a side of roasted vegetables or, for those of you on the Yellow plan, serve them on a bed of gluten-free pasta with Fresh Tomato Sauce (page 208). If you want to try something out of the ordinary, go with a blend of ground pork and lamb instead of the ground beef—or, if you're counting calories, substitute lean ground turkey for a low-fat option. No matter how you prepare them, these meatballs make for a satisfying meal.

12 ounces lean ground beef
2 large eggs, lightly beaten
½ cup almond flour
1 tablespoon chopped fresh oregano
1 tablespoon minced garlic
1 teaspoon coarse salt
½ teaspoon freshly ground black pepper
¾ cup grated Pecorino Romano cheese
3 tablespoons extra-virgin olive oil

1. In a large mixing bowl, stir together the ground beef, eggs, flour, oregano, garlic, salt, pepper, and cheese until well combined.

2. Shape the mixture into 12 meatballs and set aside on a plate.

3. In a large skillet, heat the oil over medium-high heat.

4. Add the meatballs and cook for 10 to 15 minutes, turning every 2 minutes, until evenly browned and cooked through.

NUTRITION INFO Calories 476, Total Fat 32g, Carbohydrates 4g, Protein 44g, Cholesterol 213mg

Ground Beef Casserole with Cheese Crust

SERVES 4   PREP TIME: 25 MINUTES   COOK TIME: 15 MINUTES
MEAL PLAN

Similar to a shepherd's pie, this ground beef casserole is topped with a crispy crust made from three different types of cheese. This dish has all of the components of a well-rounded meal in one recipe—tender ground beef, tasty vegetables, and a crispy cheese crust.

- 8 ounces lean ground beef
- 1 garlic clove, minced
- ½ cup diced yellow onion
- ½ teaspoon coarse salt
- ½ (12-ounce) jar roasted red peppers, drained and chopped
- 1 cup frozen peas
- ¼ teaspoon freshly ground black pepper
- ¾ cup shredded Gruyère, Parmesan, and Pecorino Romano cheese

1. Preheat the oven to 400°F.

2. In a large skillet, heat the ground beef over medium-high heat. Cook for 5 minutes or so, stirring often, until evenly browned.

3. Stir in the garlic, onion, and salt and cook for another 5 minutes.

4. Add the red peppers, frozen peas, and black pepper, then stir well and cook for 10 minutes, stirring occasionally.

5. Transfer the mixture to 2 small baking dishes and top with the Gruyère, Parmesan, and Pecorino Romano cheeses. Bake for 15 minutes or until the cheese is lightly browned and bubbling.

6. Remove the casserole from the oven and slice to serve.

NUTRITION INFO Calories 318, Total Fat 15g, Carbohydrates 11g, Protein 33g, Cholesterol 95mg

Turkey Meatloaf

SERVES 2 TO 4   PREP TIME: 10 MINUTES   COOK TIME: 40 MINUTES
MEAL PLAN

Meatloaf is the classic comfort food. Ground turkey makes a lighter meatloaf, but you won't sacrifice flavor, especially when you add some mushrooms, balsamic, and fresh thyme. The other secret to this moist meatloaf is gluten-free rolled oats.

Cooking spray
1 pound ground turkey (95 percent lean)
½ cup finely chopped onion
½ cup finely chopped mushrooms
½ cup gluten-free rolled oats
1 egg, beaten
1 tablespoon balsamic vinegar
½ teaspoon coarse salt
¼ teaspoon freshly ground black pepper

1. Preheat oven to 400°F.

2. Spray a loaf pan with nonstick cooking spray.

3. In a large bowl, combine turkey, onion, mushrooms, oats, egg, vinegar, salt, and pepper.

4. With clean hands, mix gently, just long enough to combine the ingredients well.

5. Transfer the mixture to the prepared pan and gently pat to make an even layer.

6. Bake for 40 minutes, or until a meat thermometer reaches 160°F.

7. Allow to rest for 10 minutes before slicing.

NUTRITION INFO Calories 585, Total Fat 29g, Carbohydrates 20g, Protein 69g, Cholesterol 313mg

Asian Chicken Kebabs

SERVES 2   PREP TIME: 10 MINUTES, PLUS 20 MINUTES TO MARINATE
COOK TIME: 15 MINUTES
MEAL PLAN ○ ○ ●

Sometimes food just tastes better on a stick. This Asian-inspired marinade is also delicious on veggies and fish. If using wooden skewers, soak in water for at least one hour before grilling.

1 tablespoon coconut oil, melted
2 tablespoons coconut aminos
¼ cup chicken broth
1 teaspoon grated fresh ginger
2 tablespoons finely chopped cilantro
8 ounces boneless, skinless chicken breast, cubed

1. In a large bowl, stir together the melted coconut oil, coconut aminos, chicken broth, ginger, and cilantro.

2. Add the chicken to the bowl, cover, and refrigerate for 20 minutes or up to 24 hours.

3. Preheat a grill or grill pan to medium-high heat.

4. Remove the chicken from the bowl and discard the marinade.

5. Thread the chicken on skewers and grill for 2 to 3 minutes per side, until cooked through.

6. Serve the chicken on the skewers.

NUTRITION INFO Calories 264, Total Fat 11g, Carbohydrates 2g, Protein 39g, Cholesterol 97mg

TIP Make veggie kebabs to serve along with this chicken, but be sure to keep all the veggie skewers separate. If you combine vegetables and meat on the same skewer, you will end up burning the vegetables in order to cook the chicken all the way through.

Slow-Cooker Pot Roast

SERVES 4   PREP TIME: 15 MINUTES   COOK TIME: 8 HOURS
MEAL PLAN ○ ○ ●

There is no better way to make a pot roast. After a quick pan sear, pop the ingredients into the slow cooker and your work is done. Cook on low for 8 hours, or cook on high and dinner will be ready in half the time.

1 (1½- to 2-pound) boneless chuck roast
1 teaspoon kosher salt
½ teaspoon freshly ground black pepper
1 teaspoon paprika
1 tablespoon coconut oil
1 onion, thinly sliced
1 garlic clove, minced
1 cup chicken or beef broth
1 (28-ounce) can crushed tomatoes
1 bay leaf
½ pound carrots, roughly chopped
1 fennel bulb, sliced

1. Season the meat on all sides with the salt, pepper, and paprika.

2. In a large skillet, heat the oil and sear the roast on all sides until browned.

3. Place the roast in a slow cooker.

4. Add the onion, garlic, broth, tomatoes, bay leaf, carrots, and fennel.

5. Cook on low for 8 hours.

6. Remove from the slow cooker and serve.

NUTRITION INFO Calories 563, Total Fat 22g, Carbohydrates 29g, Protein 61g, Cholesterol 129mg

Chicken Sausage Patties

SERVES 2   PREP TIME: 10 MINUTES   COOK TIME: 20 MINUTES
MEAL PLAN ○ ○ ●

It is difficult to find chicken sausage made without added sugar, so make your own (better-tasting) patties. The rice vinegar and lemon really add depth to this recipe. Serve with the Arugula and White Bean Salad (page 115) or the Balsamic Quinoa-Spinach Salad (page 110), or in a gluten-free wrap with sautéed onions and peppers.

8 ounces ground chicken
1 teaspoon ground fennel seed
½ teaspoon dried thyme
½ teaspoon coarse salt
½ teaspoon freshly ground black pepper
1 garlic clove, minced
1 teaspoon rice vinegar
½ teaspoon lemon zest
4 teaspoons extra-virgin olive oil, divided

1. In a large bowl, combine the ground chicken, fennel, thyme, salt, pepper, garlic, vinegar, and lemon zest.

2. With clean hands, mix well and shape into four patties.

3. Heat two teaspoons of oil in a large skillet over medium heat.

4. Place two patties in the pan and cook for 5 minutes per side, or until completely cooked through.

5. Repeat with the remaining oil and patties.

6. Serve as is, in a wrap, or with a salad.

NUTRITION INFO Calories 302, Total Fat 18g, Carbohydrates 1g, Protein 33g, Cholesterol 101mg

Pesto Grilled Chicken Thighs

SERVES 2   PREP TIME: 5 MINUTES   COOK TIME: 15 MINUTES
MEAL PLAN ● ● ●

Pesto is a wonderful ingredient! It is a creative way to boost flavor in pasta dishes, soups, and salad dressings, plus it makes a flavorful marinade all by itself. It is so easy to make your own, and you can store leftovers in the freezer for up to 3 months. You could also pick up a container of store-bought pesto at your local grocery store or gourmet market to save time—just check the ingredient list and make sure there are no added sweeteners.

FOR THE BASIL PESTO

3 cups fresh basil

1 clove garlic, chopped

¼ cup toasted pine nuts

Juice and zest of ½ lemon

¾ teaspoon coarse salt

¼ teaspoon black pepper

½ cup extra virgin olive oil

FOR THE CHICKEN THIGHS

¼ cup basil pesto

12 ounces boneless (skin on) chicken thighs

To make the basil pesto

1. In a food processor fitted with a steel blade, combine the basil, garlic, pine nuts, lemon juice, zest, salt, and pepper.

2. Pulse until ingredients are well chopped.

3. With the machine on, slowly pour in the olive oil.

4. Continue to blend until smooth.

To make the chicken thighs

1. Heat the grill or grill pan to medium-high.

2. In a large bowl, toss the pesto and chicken thighs until the chicken is well coated.

3. Cook, skin-side down, for 5 to 6 minutes. Turn over and cook for an additional 5 minutes, or until cooked through.

4. Allow to rest for 5 to 10 minutes before serving.

NUTRITION INFO Calories 320, Total Fat 23g, Carbohydrates 0g, Protein 26g, Cholesterol 122mg

TWELVE

AFTER-DINNER TREATS

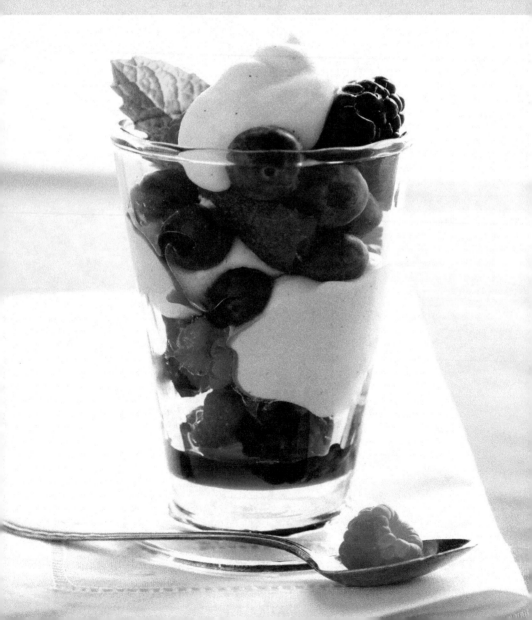

Chocolate Mousse *192*

Strawberry-Banana Cream Tart *193*

Berry–Coconut Cream Parfaits *195*

Blackberry Shooters *196*

Cucumber-Lime Refreshers *197*

Berry-Banana Dreams *198*

Marinated Bocconcini *199*

The Cheese Course *200*

Hawaiian Ice *201*

"Almond Joy" Trail Mix *202*

Chocolate-Almond Fondue *203*

Chocolate Mousse

SERVES 4   PREP TIME: 10 MINUTES
MEAL PLAN ● ○ ○ ●

This chocolate "mousse" is all you could ask for in a dessert—gluten-free, dairy-free, and full of delicious chocolate flavor. Avocado has a naturally creamy texture that whips up nicely into a mousse-like consistency. In this recipe, the use of avocado negates the need for dairy ingredients like whipping cream, which would typically be used to make the mousse.

2 large ripe avocados, pitted and chopped
2 green-tipped bananas, peeled and chopped
½ cup unsweetened cocoa powder
½ cup unsweetened coconut milk
1 teaspoon pure vanilla extract
½ teaspoon ground cinnamon
Pinch of coarse salt

1. In a food processor, combine the avocados, bananas, cocoa powder, coconut milk, vanilla, cinnamon, and salt and blend until smooth.

2. Spoon the mousse into glasses and chill until ready to serve.

NUTRITION INFO Calories 355, Total Fat 28g, Carbohydrates 30g, Protein 5g, Cholesterol 0mg

TIP It's not necessary to use canned coconut milk for this recipe. You can find unsweetened coconut milk in cartons in the dairy section at your local grocery store. Keep in mind that some companies offer flavored options, so select the "original" or "unflavored" option.

Strawberry-Banana Cream Tart

SERVES 6   PREP TIME: 15 MINUTES   COOK TIME: 35 MINUTES
MEAL PLAN ● ○ ○ ●

If you've ever made a fruit tart, you likely spent an hour or more building the crust in the pan and then whipping the filling to the right consistency. This Strawberry-Banana Cream Tart is unique in a number of ways, mainly because it's very easy to make—simply throw together the crust and combine the filling ingredients in the food processor to puree them. Green-tipped bananas impart a lightly sweet flavor as well as a creamy texture, resulting in a delectable dessert that you don't have to feel guilty about enjoying.

FOR THE CRUST

- 1½ cups almond flour
- 1 teaspoon ground cinnamon
- ¼ teaspoon coarse salt
- ¼ cup coconut oil, melted

FOR THE FILLING

- 2 green-tipped bananas, peeled and chopped
- 1 tablespoon freshly squeezed lemon juice
- 1 teaspoon vanilla extract
- 3 large eggs, lightly beaten
- ⅔ cup full-fat canned coconut milk
- 2 cups sliced fresh strawberries

To make the crust

1. Preheat the oven to 350°F.

2. In a medium mixing bowl, stir together the almond flour, cinnamon, and salt.

3. Whisk in the melted oil, then press the mixture into a pie plate, spreading it evenly along the bottom and sides. ▶

To make the filling

1. In a food processor, combine the bananas, lemon juice, vanilla, eggs, and coconut milk and blend until smooth.

2. Pour the filling into the crust and spread evenly.

3. Bake for 35 minutes, or until the center is set.

4. Cool the pie completely, then arrange the strawberries on top and slice to serve.

NUTRITION INFO Calories 277, Total Fat 23g, Carbohydrates 17g, Protein 6g, Cholesterol 93mg

TIP In following these instructions, you may find that the crust for your tart is still fairly soft. If you prefer a crisper crust, try baking the crust for 5 minutes before you add the filling.

Berry–Coconut Cream Parfaits

Made with only a handful of ingredients, these parfaits look like a gourmet dessert. If you like, sprinkle a little ground cinnamon or unsweetened cocoa powder on top to finish the presentation. Keep in mind that, when you refrigerate your cans of coconut milk, the liquid will rise to the top. To make it easier to get at the coconut cream, store the cans in the refrigerator upside down—that way you can open them from the top and scoop out the cream directly.

2 cups fresh diced strawberries
1 cup fresh blackberries
1 cup fresh blueberries
Juice of 2 lemons
2 (15-ounce) cans full-fat coconut milk,
   refrigerated overnight
2 teaspoons vanilla extract
1 teaspoon ground cinnamon
Pinch of ground cardamom

1. In a large bowl, combine the strawberries, blackberries, blueberries, and lemon juice and toss well.

2. Open the cans of coconut milk and spoon off the thick white cream into a mixing bowl. Reserve the rest of the milk in the refrigerator for another use.

3. Beat the cream with the vanilla, cinnamon, and cardamom using an electric mixer until light and fluffy, about 3 to 4 minutes.

4. Layer the berry mixture and the coconut cream in dessert glasses, then chill until ready to serve.

NUTRITION INFO Calories 262, Total Fat 20g, Carbohydrates 19g, Protein 3g, Cholesterol 9mg

Blackberry Shooters

SERVES 4   PREP TIME: 5 MINUTES, PLUS I HOUR TO REFRIGERATE
MEAL PLAN ● ○ ○ ●

This concoction made from frozen blackberries and coconut milk is so sweet and satisfying. In five minutes or less, you can prepare this delicious dessert and then store the extras in the refrigerator for later, when you're in need of a quick snack or a refreshing treat. These Blackberry Shooters are perfect to enjoy on a hot summer day after lounging by the pool, or simply as a way to refresh your mind and your palate after a long day at work. Feel free to experiment with this recipe a bit, substituting blueberries or strawberries for the blackberries.

2 cups frozen blackberries
1 cup full-fat canned coconut milk
1 tablespoon freshly squeezed lemon juice
2 or 3 ice cubes

1. In a food processor, combine the blackberries, coconut milk, lemon juice, and ice cubes.

2. Blend until smooth and well combined.

3. Pour into shot glasses, then chill in the refrigerator for at least 1 hour before serving.

NUTRITION INFO Calories 140, Total Fat 11g, Carbohydrates 9g, Protein 2g, Cholesterol 5mg

TIP If you don't have any frozen blackberries on hand, you can use fresh blackberries instead. Keep in mind that your recipe won't be as thick if you use fresh berries, however, so you may need to add a few extra ice cubes.

Cucumber-Lime Refreshers

SERVES 2 PREP TIME: 5 MINUTES
MEAL PLAN ● ● ● ●

Cucumber may not be the first ingredient that comes to mind when you think about dessert, but in this recipe it's so cool and refreshing that you might just start to think of it that way. In addition to its cool flavor, cucumber is also known for being rich in dietary fiber and other nutrients. A single 1-cup serving of cucumber contains nearly 20 percent of your daily value for vitamin K as well as plenty of pantothenic acid, copper, potassium, and manganese. Cucumbers are also full of antioxidants, which help reduce inflammation and protect the body against free-radical damage.

1 large English cucumber, peeled and diced
½ ripe avocado, pitted and chopped
Juice of 1 lime
2 tablespoons ground flaxseed
2 tablespoons chia seeds
2 or 3 ice cubes

1. In a food processor, combine the cucumber, avocado, lime juice, flaxseed, chia seeds, and ice cubes and blend until smooth.

2. Pour into glasses and serve immediately.

NUTRITION INFO Calories 191, Total Fat 15g, Carbohydrates 15g, Protein 5g, Cholesterol 0mg

Berry-Banana Dreams

SERVES I   PREP TIME: 5 MINUTES
MEAL PLAN ● ◐ ◌

Cool and creamy, these fruity treats are the perfect way to top off a tasty meal. By using green-tipped bananas in this recipe, you'll get a lightly sweet flavor that's all natural—no added sugar required. Feel free to use whatever berries you have on hand for this recipe, and keep in mind that frozen berries work, too, as long as you thaw them first. Don't be afraid to mix it up with a combination of blueberries, blackberries, and strawberries, or simply pick your favorite.

½ cup fresh berries (your choice)
1 cup plain Greek yogurt
1 small green-tipped banana, peeled and sliced
1 ice cube

1. In a blender, combine the berries, yogurt, banana, and ice cube.

2. Blend on high speed until smooth, then pour into a glass and serve.

NUTRITION INFO Calories 350, Total Fat 15g, Carbohydrates 47g, Protein 11g, Cholesterol 50mg

TIP To enjoy this recipe on the Blue meal plan, all you have to do is replace the Greek yogurt with a nondairy alternative. Full-fat canned coconut milk will give this recipe the thickness it needs without adding any dairy.

Marinated Bocconcini

SERVES 4   PREP TIME: 10 MINUTES, PLUS 4 HOURS TO REFRIGERATE
MEAL PLAN ● ◐ ◌

Bocconcini are small balls of fresh mozzarella cheese, typically about the size of an egg. These cheeses are semisoft and mild, which makes them perfect for snacking. In fact, the name bocconcini is derived from the Italian for "small mouthfuls." Today, most bocconcini is made from a combination of cow's milk and water buffalo milk, which is why it is sometimes called uova di bufala—"buffalo eggs." If you can't find fresh bocconcini at your local grocery store, check an Italian supermarket or a specialty foods store.

1 pound drained bocconcini
¾ cup extra-virgin olive oil
2 tablespoons drained capers, chopped
2 tablespoons chopped fresh parsley
1 tablespoon chopped fresh thyme
1 teaspoon crushed red pepper flakes
1 teaspoon minced garlic
1 teaspoon coarse salt

1. In a large mixing bowl, toss the bocconcini with the oil until well coated.

2. Add the capers, parsley, thyme, red pepper, garlic, and salt, and toss well to coat.

3. Transfer to an airtight container, then chill for 4 hours before serving.

NUTRITION INFO Calories 259, Total Fat 20g, Carbohydrates 1g, Protein 25g, Cholesterol 61mg

The Cheese Course

SERVES 4 TO 6   PREP TIME: 5 MINUTES
MEAL PLAN ● ◉ ◉

The cheese course is typically part of a multicourse meal, usually served after the main dish and before dessert. For cheese lovers, any meal without cheese could be considered incomplete. A nineteenth-century French aphorism states, "Un dessert sans fromage est une belle à qui il manque un œil"—a dessert without cheese is a one-eyed beauty. If you're curious about instituting a cheese course in your own dietary routine, this recipe is the perfect place to start. Feel free to substitute different kinds of cheeses for those mentioned in the recipe; all that matters is that you have a variety.

1 large piece hard Asiago cheese
1 small soft Brie
1 recipe Lemon-Marinated Olives (page 98)
1 recipe Marinated Bocconcini (page 199)
1 cup raw almonds
1 cup fresh blackberries

1. Arrange the cheeses on a platter, and place the marinated olives and bocconcini in bowls.

2. Scatter the raw almonds and blackberries over the platter to enhance the presentation.

3. Serve with cheese knives and appetizer plates.

NUTRITION INFO Calories 581, Total Fat 46g, Carbohydrates 12g, Protein 29g, Cholesterol 77mg

TIP This recipe gives you the perfect reason to check out the artisanal cheese section at your local grocery store or specialty food store. Don't be afraid to try something new! Most places are happy to give you a sample of several cheeses, so try a few before deciding what you want to buy.

Hawaiian Ice

SERVES 2   PREP TIME: 20 MINUTES, PLUS 12 HOURS TO FREEZE
MEAL PLAN   ● ○ ○ ○

Also known simply as shave ice, Hawaiian ice is a treat that originated in Japan during the Heian period. When Japanese plantation workers immigrated to the Hawaiian Islands, they brought their tradition of shave ice with them. You can simply shave the ice using a grater. Don't be afraid to try different things, like almond milk with your Hawaiian Ice instead of coconut milk.

Cooking spray
Water
¼ cup unsweetened coconut milk

1. Lightly grease the inside of a loaf pan with cooking spray and fill it with water.

2. Place the pan in the freezer and freeze overnight, or until solid.

3. Turn the block of ice out onto a solid surface and carefully grate it using a hand grater.

4. Grate the ice until you have about 2 cups, then divide between two dessert glasses.

5. Drizzle the coconut milk over the ice to serve.

NUTRITION INFO Calories 71, Total Fat 7g, Carbohydrates 2g, Protein 1g, Cholesterol 0mg

TIP It can take several hours for a large block of ice to freeze, so be sure to give yourself plenty of time—place the water-filled loaf pan in the freezer at least 12 hours ahead of time. Another option is to freeze two smaller containers of water that may not require as much time.

"Almond Joy" Trail Mix

YIELDS ABOUT 3 CUPS   PREP TIME: 5 MINUTES   COOK TIME: 15 MINUTES   MEAL PLAN ● ● ● ●

While Almond Joy candy bars are definitely not allowed on the sugar detox, that doesn't mean you can't enjoy all of the flavors you would find in the candy bar. This recipe combines the taste of crunchy almonds with tender coconut and just a hint of salt. Take this trail mix with you as you run your daily errands to ensure that you never go hungry and that you don't succumb to the temptation to go off the detox. If you have a tasty snack option right in your bag, you will be less tempted to stray!

2 cups raw almonds
2 tablespoons extra-virgin olive oil
Coarse salt
1 cup shredded unsweetened coconut

1. Preheat the oven to 300°F.

2. In a large mixing bowl, toss the almonds with the oil and season with salt.

3. Spread the almonds evenly on a rimmed baking sheet. Bake for 10 minutes, until lightly toasted.

4. Sprinkle the coconut over the almonds and bake for another 5 minutes, until the coconut is just browned.

5. Remove from the oven and cool completely.

6. Serve at room temperature, and store leftovers in an airtight container.

NUTRITION INFO (½ cup), Calories 270, Total Fat 25g, Carbohydrates 9g, Protein 7g, Cholesterol 0mg

Chocolate-Almond Fondue

SERVES 2　PREP TIME: 10 MINUTES　COOK TIME: 1 TO 2 MINUTES
MEAL PLAN　● ● ● ●

A fresh, healthy take on a sugar-laden treat—here is a dip you can feel good about eating. From the antioxidants in the chocolate to the vitamin E in the almonds and the fiber in the fruit, this simple recipe packs more than delicious flavor. Serve on a platter with toothpicks for easy dipping.

¼ cup almond butter

1 teaspoon unsweetened cocoa powder

3 tablespoons canned coconut milk

1 green-tipped banana, sliced

1 cup strawberries, sliced

1. In a small, microwave-safe dish, stir together the almond butter, cocoa, and coconut milk until well combined.

2. Place in the microwave and cook on high for 30 seconds.

3. Remove from the microwave, stir again, and place back in the microwave for 30 seconds more. Repeat until the mixture is warm and gooey.

4. Serve with the bananas and strawberries for dipping.

NUTRITION INFO Calories 328, Total Fat 24g, Carbohydrates 26g, Protein 8g, Cholesterol 0mg

THIRTEEN

CONDIMENTS, DRESSINGS & SAUCES

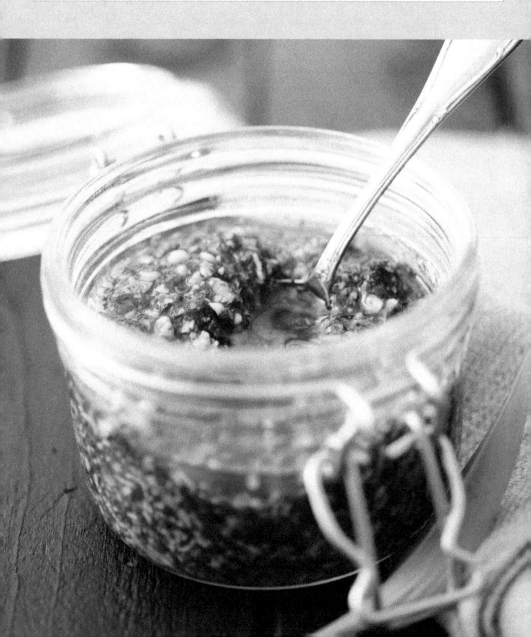

Mayonnaise 206

Au Jus 207

Fresh Tomato Sauce 208

Blue Cheese Dressing 210

Green Goddess Dressing 211

Pico de Gallo 212

Chimichurri Sauce 213

Fresh Pickled Vegetables 214

Fresh Pesto Sauce 215

No-Cook White Sauce 216

Mint Tzatziki 217

Mayonnaise

YIELDS ABOUT 2 CUPS   PREP TIME: 10 MINUTES
MEAL PLAN ● ○ ○ ○ ●

Mayonnaise, a thick French sauce, is often used as a condiment on sandwiches and as an ingredient in salads and dressings. Unfortunately, many commercially produced mayonnaise products contain sugar and other ingredients that make them a "no" food for the sugar detox. Luckily, this recipe makes it easy to prepare your own mayonnaise using all-natural ingredients. With little more than egg yolks, olive oil, and vinegar, you can create a creamy, sugar-free mayonnaise to use in all your favorite sugar detox recipes throughout this book.

2 large egg yolks
¼ cup red wine vinegar
1 tablespoon Dijon mustard
1½ cups extra-virgin olive oil
Coarse salt

1. In a food processor, combine the egg yolks, vinegar, and mustard.

2. Blend until smooth and well combined.

3. With the processor running, drizzle in the oil in a steady stream. Season with salt to taste.

4. Store in the refrigerator for up to five days.

PER SERVING (1 tablespoon): Calories 85, Total Fat 10g, Carbohydrates 0g, Protein 0g, Cholesterol 13mg

Au Jus

YIELD ABOUT I CUP   PREP TIME: 5 MINUTES   COOK TIME: I0 MINUTES
MEAL PLAN ● ● ●

Au jus is a French term meaning "in its own juice." This au jus can be made from any meat that has been baked or roasted in the oven—simply reserve the juice and the bits of meat sticking to the pan and use them to prepare this recipe. If you're making au jus from chicken or turkey, use chicken broth; for beef, pork, or lamb, use beef broth.

Roasting pan with meat juice, meat removed
½ cup water
1 cup low-sodium beef or chicken broth
1 tablespoon chopped fresh parsley
2 tablespoons coconut oil

1. Heat the pan in which you cooked the meat over high heat and pour in the water. Stir the water around to loosen the bits of meat and fat stuck to the pan.

2. Add the broth to the pan and continue to stir until it comes to a simmer.

3. Stir in the parsley and oil, stirring until the oil melts and the liquid is very hot.

4. Serve the au jus over the cooked meat.

NUTRITION INFO Calories 69, Total Fat 7g, Carbohydrates 0g, Protein 1g, Cholesterol 0mg

Fresh Tomato Sauce

YIELDS ABOUT 12 CUPS   PREP TIME: 15 MINUTES   COOK TIME: 45 MINUTES
MEAL PLAN ● ● ● ●

You may be wondering why tomato sauce is a recipe in this book when it's such an easy product to find at the grocery store. What you may not realize, however, is that most commercially produced tomato sauces contain several grams of sugar per serving. In these products, sugar is used to cut the acid of the tomatoes, as they are stored on the shelf for long periods of time. But in making your own tomato sauce, you don't have to worry about that. Feel free to dress up the sauce by adding a handful of your favorite herbs, such as basil, parsley, or fresh oregano.

4 pounds ripe tomatoes
⅓ cup extra-virgin olive oil
1 large yellow onion, diced
1 tablespoon minced garlic
1 medium carrot, peeled and diced
1 large celery stalk, diced
Salt
Freshly ground black pepper

1. Bring a large pot of water to a boil over high heat.

2. Use a sharp knife to slice an "X" into the top of each tomato, then place them in the boiling water in batches for 10 to 15 seconds each.

3. Remove the tomatoes with a slotted spoon and remove the skin. Chop the tomatoes and set aside.

4. In a large skillet, heat the oil, then add the onion and garlic. Cook for 5 minutes, stirring occasionally, until the onion is translucent.

5. Stir in the carrot and celery and cook for 5 minutes more, stirring occasionally.

6. Add the tomatoes and season with salt and pepper. Reduce the heat and simmer for 45 minutes, until the tomatoes have broken down.

7. Remove the skillet from the heat and stir in some water, if needed, to thin the sauce. Adjust the seasonings as needed.

PER SERVING (1 cup): Calories 96, Total Fat 7g, Carbohydrates 8g, Protein 2g, Cholesterol 0mg

TIP If you know that you're going to be using tomato sauce in one of the recipes in this book, try to make this sauce ahead of time so it will be ready to use. It can easily be stored in the refrigerator for up to a week.

Blue Cheese Dressing

YIELDS ABOUT 2 CUPS   PREP TIME: 5 MINUTES
MEAL PLAN ● ◐ ◐

If you're a fan of thick and creamy salad dressings, this Blue Cheese Dressing is for you. Adding a dollop to your salad will make you feel less like you're sacrificing a heartier meal option for the sake of health; this dressing turns even the plainest salad into a delicious indulgence. Made with your homemade Mayonnaise recipe from this book, along with Greek yogurt, this dressing is cool and creamy, flavored with garlic and blue cheese crumbles. Don't be afraid to try this dressing on dishes other than salads—it also makes a tasty topping for grilled chicken.

1 cup Mayonnaise (page 206)
½ cup plain Greek yogurt
1 tablespoon minced yellow onion
1 tablespoon minced garlic
1 tablespoon freshly squeezed lemon juice
1 tablespoon distilled white vinegar
½ cup blue cheese crumbles
Salt
Freshly ground black pepper

1. In a food processor, combine the Mayonnaise, Greek yogurt, onion, garlic, lemon juice, vinegar, and cheese. Season with salt and pepper.

2. Blend on high speed for 20 to 40 seconds until smooth.

3. Store in an airtight container in the refrigerator for up to a week.

PER SERVING (2 tablespoons): Calories 78, Total Fat 6g, Carbohydrates 5g, Protein 1g, Cholesterol 10mg

Green Goddess Dressing

YIELDS ABOUT 2 CUPS   PREP TIME: 5 MINUTES
MEAL PLAN ◌ ◌ ●

If you go to the grocery store for salad dressing, you will find hundreds of different options. Though all of these options may vary in flavor, many of them have one thing in common—they contain sugar and artificial ingredients. As you will find in reading this book, salads are a great food to enjoy on the sugar detox because they are naturally sugar-free and full of nutrients. If you're going to be eating a lot of salads, you need a tasty dressing to go with them, and this Green Goddess Dressing certainly fits the bill!

1 cup Mayonnaise (page 206)
1 ripe avocado, pitted and chopped
4 anchovy fillets, rinsed and diced
2 tablespoons sliced scallions
2 tablespoons chopped fresh parsley
1 tablespoon freshly squeezed lemon juice
1 teaspoon minced garlic
Salt
Freshly ground black pepper

1. In a food processor, combine the Mayonnaise, avocado, anchovies, scallions, parsley, lemon juice, and garlic. Season with salt and pepper.

2. Blend on high speed for 20 to 40 seconds until smooth.

3. Store in an airtight container in the refrigerator for up to a week.

PER SERVING (2 tablespoons): Calories 86, Total Fat 8g, Carbohydrates 5g, Protein 1g, Cholesterol 5mg

Pico de Gallo

YIELDS ABOUT 2 CUPS   PREP TIME: 10 MINUTES
MEAL PLAN ● ○ ○ ○

Though the term pico de gallo *means "rooster's beak" in Spanish, it's a dish that has nothing to do with chicken—unless, of course, you serve it on top of chicken. This side dish is also called salsa fresca because it's a kind of fresh salsa made from chopped tomatoes, peppers, and onions. Serve your Pico de Gallo with your favorite Mexican dish or as a topping for grilled chicken or fish. If you have it available, feel free to add chopped fresh cilantro.*

3 large ripe tomatoes, cored and diced
1 small sweet onion, diced
1 jalapeño pepper, seeded and minced
2 garlic cloves, minced
3 scallions, sliced
Juice of 1 lime
Salt
Freshly ground black pepper

1. In a medium mixing bowl, stir together the tomatoes, onion, jalapeño, garlic, and scallions.

2. Toss with the lime juice and season with salt and pepper to taste.

PER SERVING (½ cup): Calories 39, Total Fat 0g, Carbohydrates 9g, Protein 2g, Cholesterol 0mg

Chimichurri Sauce

YIELDS ABOUT 2 CUPS   PREP TIME: 5 MINUTES
MEAL PLAN ● ○ ○ ●

Chimichurri sauce is a type of green sauce that originated in Argentina, where it's typically used for grilled meat, though you can use it on whatever you want. Made from fresh parsley and garlic blended with olive oil and red wine vinegar, this sauce is full of flavor without being so intense that it overpowers the flavor of the meat. To make the most of this sauce, use it as a marinade before you grill your favorite meat and serve a little extra on the side.

1 cup chopped fresh parsley leaves
½ cup extra-virgin olive oil
⅓ cup red wine vinegar
¼ cup chopped fresh cilantro
Juice of ½ lemon
1 tablespoon minced garlic
1 teaspoon crushed red pepper flakes
½ teaspoon ground cumin
½ teaspoon coarse salt

1. Combine the parsley, oil, vinegar, cilantro, lemon juice, garlic, red pepper flakes, cumin, and salt in a food processor.

2. Blend on high speed for 20 to 40 seconds until smooth.

3. Store in an airtight container in the refrigerator for up to a week.

PER SERVING (¼ cup): Calories 116, Total Fat 13g, Carbohydrates 1g, Protein 0g, Cholesterol 0mg

Fresh Pickled Vegetables

YIELDS ABOUT 4 CUPS   PREP TIME: I0 MINUTES
MEAL PLAN ● ○ ○ ●

These Fresh Pickled Vegetables are a great snack to have on hand when you simply need a little something to munch on. Crisp and salty, they will soon become one of your favorite snacks. Try this recipe with all of your favorite vegetables, including carrots, onion, celery, bell peppers, and more. If you can't decide, feel free to do what the recipe suggests and go with a combination of chopped vegetables. Serve this dish as a snack between meals or as a side dish—it goes particularly well as a side for sandwiches.

4 cups mixed chopped vegetables
⅓ cup red wine vinegar
1 small sweet onion, minced
1 tablespoon minced garlic
2 teaspoons chopped fresh basil
1 teaspoon coarse salt
1 teaspoon whole peppercorns

1. Put the vegetables in a large glass jar or bowl.

2. In a small bowl, whisk together the vinegar, onion, garlic, basil, salt, and peppercorns and pour over the vegetables. Toss to coat.

3. Cover and chill for 24 hours before serving.

4. Store in the refrigerator for up to a week.

PER SERVING (½ cup): Calories 62, Total Fat 0g, Carbohydrates 13g, Protein 3g, Cholesterol 0mg

Fresh Pesto Sauce

YIELDS ABOUT 2 CUPS   PREP TIME: 10 MINUTES
MEAL PLAN ● ●

Pesto is a type of Italian herb sauce traditionally made from garlic, basil, and pine nuts, with olive oil and Parmigiano-Reggiano cheese. Pesto can be used to top cooked meats or stirred into cooked pasta to provide a fresh flavor. The best part about this sauce is that it's naturally sugar-free, so you don't have to worry about this recipe being a downgrade from the original. If you're feeling adventurous, try adding some fresh cilantro to the recipe or using cilantro instead of basil entirely.

3 tablespoons toasted pine nuts
1½ cups chopped fresh basil
¼ cup freshly grated Parmigiano-Reggiano cheese
1 tablespoon minced garlic
½ teaspoon coarse salt
¼ teaspoon freshly ground black pepper
1 tablespoon freshly squeezed lemon juice
½ cup extra-virgin olive oil

1. In a small skillet, cook the pine nuts over medium heat for 3 to 4 minutes, stirring often, until lightly browned. Set the nuts aside to cool.

2. Combine the basil, cheese, toasted pine nuts, garlic, salt, pepper, and lemon juice in a food processor.

3. Blend on high speed until the mixture is smooth and well combined.

4. With the processor running, drizzle in the oil to form a thick paste. Adjust seasonings as needed.

5. Store in the refrigerator for up to a week.

PER SERVING (2 tablespoons): Calories 78, Total Fat 8g, Carbohydrates 1g, Protein 2g, Cholesterol 3mg

No-Cook White Sauce

YIELDS ABOUT 1 CUP   PREP TIME: 5 MINUTES
MEAL PLAN ● ○ ○ ○ ●

Want to dress up a grilled chicken breast or a piece of fish? Try this simple white sauce. Since it's made with your own homemade Mayonnaise from this book, you can rest assured that it's entirely sugar-free and contains only healthy ingredients. If you were to buy white sauce at the grocery store, it would likely be loaded with sugar, flour, and artificial preservatives. In this recipe, however, you will find nothing more than Mayonnaise, vinegar, lemon juice, and seasonings. Keep a jar of this sauce handy for whenever you serve chicken or fish.

½ cup Mayonnaise (page 216)
1 tablespoon distilled white vinegar
2 teaspoons freshly squeezed lemon juice
1 teaspoon coarse salt
1 teaspoon freshly ground pepper
1 teaspoon minced garlic

1. Combine the Mayonnaise, vinegar, lemon juice, salt, pepper, and garlic in a food processor.

2. Blend on high speed for 20 to 40 seconds until smooth.

3. Store in the refrigerator for up to a week.

PER SERVING (¼ cup): Calories 118, Total Fat 10g, Carbohydrates 8g, Protein 0g, Cholesterol 8mg

Mint Tzatziki

YIELDS 1¼ CUPS   PREP TIME: 10 MINUTES, PLUS 20 MINUTES TO CHILL
MEAL PLAN ● ○ ○

It is hard to believe a combo of such simple ingredients can taste so amazing. Use this sauce as a dip for fresh vegetables or as a condiment for cooked meats, fish, or vegetables. This cool, creamy Greek dish will bring a unique spin to whatever you pair it with.

1 cup low-fat Greek yogurt
½ large English cucumber, finely chopped
1 garlic clove, finely chopped
2 teaspoons distilled white vinegar
1 tablespoon fresh chopped mint
½ teaspoon kosher salt

1. In a medium bowl, stir together the yogurt, cucumber, garlic, and vinegar.

2. Add the mint and salt and stir again.

3. Cover and allow to chill in the refrigerator for 20 minutes before serving.

PER SERVING (¼ cup): Calories 59, Total Fat 1g, Carbohydrates 12g, Protein 2g, Cholesterol 2mg

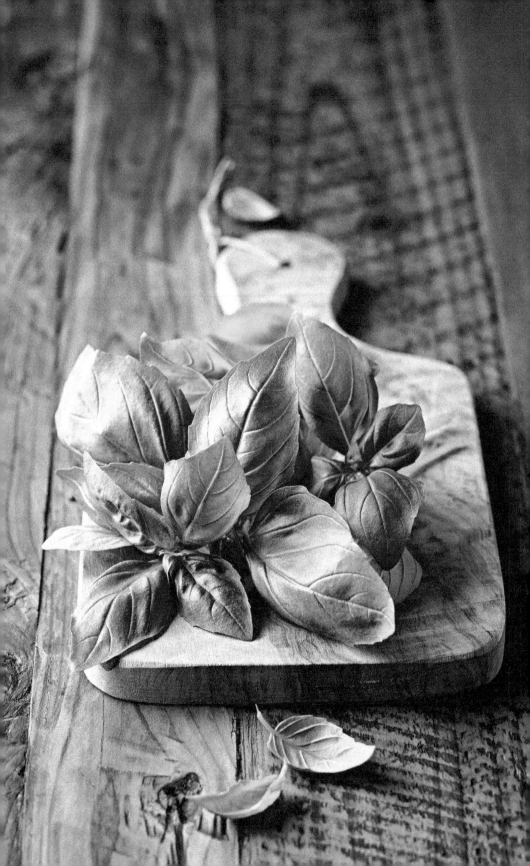

RESOURCES

If you're not used to the dietary restrictions in the various sugar detox plans, you may have a little difficulty adjusting. For example, it may take you some time to learn your way around the organic and natural sections of your grocery store. If you're having trouble finding an unfamiliar ingredient for one of the recipes in this book, the natural food section at your grocery store is a good place to start. If your grocery store doesn't have the item in stock, try your local health food store or look into online retailers. When scanning the aisles, keep these recommended brands in mind:

- Applegate Farms: bacon, sausage, and deli meats
- Artisana: coconut oil, coconut butter, and other products
- Coconut Secret: coconut aminos (a great substitute for soy sauce)
- Eden Foods: wide range of organic products
- Once Again: organic nut butters
- Penzeys Spices: herbs and spices of all kinds; also available online at Penzeys.com
- Silk: dairy-free milk products such as almond milk, coconut milk, etc.
- Simply Organics: wide range of products
- Thai Kitchen: coconut milk
- U.S. Wellness Meats: meats, eggs, and meat snacks

If your local grocery stores have a limited selection, or if you simply can't find the right quantity of ingredients you use often, you may want to consider buying online. The following is a list of excellent online resources for some of the most commonly used ingredients in the recipes in this book.

- Alive and Radiant Foods (EatAliveandRadiant.com): a company that makes a variety of snacks, including dehydrated kale chips

- Amazon (Amazon.com): a one-stop shop that offers a wide range of healthy food items and supplies

- Bergin Fruit and Nut Company (BerginFruit.com): a leading supplier of nuts, dried fruit, and trail mix

- Eat Wild (EatWild.com): a great website where you can search for organic growers and suppliers in your area

- King Arthur Flour (KingArthurFlour.com): a leading supplier of organic and natural baking ingredients

- The Vegan Store (VeganStore.com): a supplier of dairy-free substitutes, including cheese and milk

MEASUREMENT CONVERSIONS

Volume Equivalents (Liquid)

U.S. STANDARD	U.S. STANDARD (OUNCES)	METRIC (APPROXIMATE)
2 tablespoons	1 fl. oz.	30 mL
¼ cup	2 fl. oz.	60 mL
½ cup	4 fl. oz.	120 mL
1 cup	8 fl. oz.	240 mL
1½ cups	12 fl. oz.	355 mL
2 cups or 1 pint	16 fl. oz.	475 mL
4 cups or 1 quart	32 fl. oz.	1 L
1 gallon	128 fl. oz.	4 L

Oven Temperatures

FAHRENHEIT (F)	CELSIUS (C) (APPROXIMATE)
250	120
300	150
325	165
350	180
375	190
400	200
425	220
450	230

Volume Equivalents (Dry)

U.S. STANDARD	METRIC (APPROXIMATE)
⅛ teaspoon	0.5 mL
¼ teaspoon	1 mL
½ teaspoon	2 mL
¾ teaspoon	4 mL
1 teaspoon	5 mL
1 tablespoon	15 mL
¼ cup	59 mL
⅓ cup	79 mL
½ cup	118 mL
⅔ cup	156 mL
¾ cup	177 mL
1 cup	235 mL
2 cups or 1 pint	475 mL
3 cups	700 mL
4 cups or 1 quart	1 L
½ gallon	2 L
1 gallon	4 L

Weight Equivalents

U.S. STANDARD	METRIC (APPROXIMATE)
½ ounce	15 g
1 ounce	30 g
2 ounces	60 g
4 ounces	115 g
8 ounces	225 g
12 ounces	340 g
16 ounces or 1 pound	455 g

REFERENCES

American Chemical Society. "Drink Water to Curb Weight Gain? Clinical Trial Confirms Effectiveness of Simple Appetite Control Method." *ScienceDaily.* Accessed May 19, 2014. www.sciencedaily.com/releases /2010/08/100823142929.htm.

American Diabetes Association. "Fast Facts: Data and Statistics About Diabetes." Accessed May 18, 2014. http://professional.diabetes.org /admin/UserFiles/0%20-%20Sean/Documents/Fast_Facts_9-2014.pdf

American Diabetes Association. "Sugar Alcohols." Accessed May 18, 2014. www.diabetes.org/food-and-fitness/food/what-can-i-eat/understanding -carbohydrates/sugar-alcohols.html.

American Heart Association. "Sugar 101." Accessed June 1, 2014. www.heart.org/HEARTORG/GettingHealthy/NutritionCenter /HealthyEating/Sugar-101_UCM_306024_Article.jsp.

Anton, Stephen D., et al. "Effects of Chromium Picolinate on Food Intake and Satiety." *Diabetes Technology & Therapeutics* 10, no. 5 (October 2008): 405–412. Accessed June 10, 2014. www.ncbi.nlm.nih.gov/pmc /articles/PMC2753428.

Aronson, Dina. "Cortisol—Its Role in Stress, Inflammation, and Indications for Diet Therapy." *Today's Dietitian* 11, no. 11 (November 2009): 38. Accessed August 29, 2014. www.todaysdietitian.com/newarchives /111609p38.shtml.

Busch, Sandi. "Good & Bad Sugars." *SFGate.* Accessed June 1, 2014. http:// healthyeating.sfgate.com/good-bad-sugars-7608.html.

Christ, Anika. "How Sugar Influences Your Sense of Taste." *LifeTime WeightLoss.* Accessed June 2, 2014. www.lifetime-weightloss.com/blog /2011/8/19/how-sugar-influences-your-sense-of-taste.html.

DeNoon, Daniel J. "Chromium May Cut Carb Craving in Depression." WebMD. Accessed May 19, 2014. www.webmd.com/depression/news /20040603/chromium-may-cut-carb-craving-in-depression.

"Effect of Legumes as Part of a Low Glycemic Index Diet on Glycemic Control and Cardiovascular Risk Factors in Type 2 Diabetes Mellitus." JAMA Network. Accessed May 19, 2014. http://archinte.jamanetwork .com/article.aspx?articleid=1384247.

Elobeid, Mai, David Brock, Miguel Padilla, and Douglas Ruden. "Endo-crine Disruptors and Obesity: An Examination of Selected Persistent Organic Pollutants in the NHANES 1999–2002 Data." *International Journal of Environmental Research Public Health* 7, no. 7 (2010): 2988–3005. Accessed December 3, 2014. http://www.ncbi.nlm.nih.gov/ pmc/articles/PMC2922741/?tool=pubmed.

Freed, David L. J. "Do Dietary Lectins Cause Disease?" *British Medical Journal* 318, no. 7190 (April 1999): 1023–1024. doi: dx.doi.org/10.1136/bmj.318.7190.1023.

Haas, Elson M. "Sugar Detox: How to Reduce Cravings and Manage Withdrawal." *Mother Earth Living.* Accessed May 19, 2014. www.motherearthliving.com/health-and-wellness/sugar-detox-sugar-withdrawal-ze0z1206zmel.aspx#ixzz31ZQKXxCd.

Hoebel, Bartley, Pedro Rada, and Nicole Avena. "Evidence for Sugar Addiction: Behavioral and Neurochemical Effects of Intermittent, Excessive Sugar Intake." *Neuroscience and Biobehavioral Reviews* 32, no. 1 (2007): 20–39. Accessed December 3, 2014. www.ncbi.nlm.nih.gov/pmc/articles/PMC2235907/.

Holmes, Philip. "UGA and Emory Awarded $1.9 Million Grant to Study How Regular Aerobic Exercise." The University of Georgia. Accessed May 19, 2014. www.news.uga.edu/releases/print/uga-and-emory-awarded-1.9-million-grant.

"Insufficient Sleep Is a Public Health Epidemic." Centers for Disease Control and Prevention. January 13, 2014. Accessed December 3, 2014. www.cdc.gov/features/dssleep/.

"Lactose Intolerance." National Institute of Diabetes and Digestive and Kidney Diseases. Accessed December 3, 2014. www.niddk.nih.gov/health-information/health-topics/digestive-diseases/lactose-intolerance/Pages/facts.aspx.

"Lactose Intolerance." *The New York Times.* Accessed May 18, 2014. www.nytimes.com/health/guides/disease/lactose-intolerance/overview.html.

"Legume and Soy Food Intake and the Incidence of Type 2 Diabetes in the Shanghai Women's Health Study." *The American Journal of Clinical Nutrition.* Accessed December 3, 2014. http://ajcn.nutrition.org/content/87/1/162.abstract.

Malik, Vasanti, Matthias Schulze, and Frank Hu. "Intake of Sugar-sweetened Beverages and Weight Gain: A Systematic Review." *American Journal of Clinical Nutrition* 84, no. 2 (2006): 274–88. Accessed December 3, 2014. www.ncbi.nlm.nih.gov/pmc/articles/PMC3210834/.

"Milk Allergy. Causes." Mayo Clinic. Accessed December 3, 2014. www.mayoclinic.org/diseases-conditions/milk-allergy/basics/causes/con-20032147.

"Milk Allergy." Food Allergy Research & Education. Accessed December 3, 2014. www.foodallergy.org/allergens/milk-allergy.

Nestle, Marion. *What to Eat.* New York: North Point Press, 2006.

Payne, A. N., et al. "Gut Microbial Adaptation to Dietary Consumption of Fructose, Artificial Sweeteners and Sugar Alcohols: Implications for Host–Microbe Interactions Contributing to Obesity." *Obesity Reviews* 13 (2012): 799–809. doi: 10.1111/j.1467-789X.2012.01009.x.

Rada, P., et al. "Abstract: Daily Bingeing on Sugar Repeatedly Releases Dopamine in the Accumbens Shell." National Center for Biotechnology Information. Accessed May 19, 2014. www.ncbi.nlm.nih.gov/pubmed/15987666.

"Recombinant Bovine Growth Hormone." American Cancer Society. Accessed December 3, 2014. www.cancer.org/cancer/cancercauses/othercarcinogens/athome/recombinant-bovine-growth-hormone.

Rensburg, Janse Van, et al. "Acute Exercise Modulates Cigarette Cravings and Brain Activation in Response to Smoking-Related Images: An fMRI Study." *Psychopharmacology* 203, no. 3 (April 2009): 589–98. Accessed June 10, 2014. www.ncbi.nlm.nih.gov/pubmed/19015835.

Sartor, Francesco, and Lucy Donaldson. "Taste Perception and Implicit Attitude Toward Sweet Related to Body Mass Index and Soft Drink Supplementation." *Appetite* 57 (2011): 237–246.

"Sleep Deprivation Linked to Junk Food Cravings." UC Berkeley News-Center. Accessed May 19, 2014. http://newscenter.berkeley.edu/2013/08/06/poor-sleep-junk-food.

Southgate, David A. T. "Digestion and Metabolism of Sugars." *The American Journal of Clinical Nutrition*. Accessed May 18, 2014. http://ajcn.nutrition.org/content/62/1/203S.full.pdf.

Srivastava, Mala. "List of Good Carbs & Bad Carbs." *SFGate*. Accessed May 19, 2014. http://healthyeating.sfgate.com/list-good-carbs-bad-carbs-6520.html.

United Nations Observances. www.un.org/en/events/observances/years.shtml. Accessed December 10, 2014.

United States Food and Drug Administration. "Guidance for Industry: A Labeling Guide (9. Appendix A: Definitions of Nutrient Content Claims)." Accessed May 19, 2014. www.fda.gov/food/guidanceregulation/guidancedocumentsregulatoryinformation/labelingnutrition/ucm064911.htm.

Ussher, M., et al. "Abstract: Effect of a Short Bout of Exercise on Tobacco Withdrawal Symptoms and Desire to Smoke." National Center for Biotechnology Information. Accessed May 19, 2014. www.ncbi.nlm.nih.gov/pubmed/11685385.

Wells, Hodan Farah, and Jean C. Buzby. "Dietary Assessment of Major Trends in U.S. Food Consumption, 1970–2005." U.S. Department of Agriculture. Accessed May 19, 2014. www.ers.usda.gov/publications/eib-economic-information-bulletin/eib33.aspx#.U3EFgV5g6Ek.

Woodruff, Cathryn. "Is Sugar from Fruit Better for You Than White Sugar?" *Huffington Post*. Accessed June 10, 2014. www.huffingtonpost.com/2013/06/29/fruit-sugar-versus-white-sugar_n_3497795.html.

RECIPE INDEX

A

"Almond Joy" Trail Mix, 202
Argentinean-Style Beef, 181
Asian Chicken Kebabs, 185
Asian Slaw with Thai Tofu,
    139–140
Asparagus and Prosciutto
    Salad, 116
Au Jus, 207

B

Bacon and Broccoli
    Salad, 108
Bacon-Wrapped Chicken
    Bites, 96
Baked Vegetable Chips, 105
Baked White Fish Fillets,
    158–159
Balsamic Quinoa-Spinach
    Salad, 110–111
Banana-Walnut Morning
    "Sundae," 76
Berry-Banana Dreams, 198
Berry-Coconut Cream
    Parfaits, 195
Blackberry Shooters, 196
Blackened Salmon with
    Cucumber Salsa,
    164–165
Blue Cheese Dressing, 210
Breakfast Grains with
    Hazelnuts, 77–78

C

The Cheese Course, 200
Cheesy Bacon Breakfast
    Casserole, 81–82
Chicken Fajita Lettuce
    Cups, 175
Chicken Salad with
    Walnuts, 109

Chicken Sausage
    Patties, 187
Chile-Lime Grilled Salmon,
    160–161
Chimichurri Sauce, 213
Chocolate-Almond
    Fondue, 203
Chocolate Blackberry
    Frappé, 70
Chocolate Mousse, 192
Cod and Green Beans in
    Parchment, 168–169
Creamy Spinach and Bacon
    Pie, 177
Crunchy Kale Chips, 94
Crustless Spring Quiche, 86
Cucumber and Tuna Salad
    Bites, 100
Cucumber-Lime
    Refreshers, 197
Curried Carrot Soup with
    Basil, 121
Curry-Ginger Pork
    Chops, 178

D

Double-Boiler Scrambled
    Eggs, 83

E

Egg and Prosciutto-Stuffed
    Mushroom Caps, 84–85
Eggplant Sandwiches with
    Herbed Feta, 124–125

F

Fresh Pesto Sauce, 215
Fresh Pickled
    Vegetables, 214
Fresh Tomato Sauce,
    208–209

G

Grain-Free Granola,
    79–80
Green Goddess Dressing, 211
Green Tea Smoothie, 72
Grilled Garlic-Rosemary
    Pork Tenderloin with
    Steamed Broccoli,
    179–180
Grilled Portobello
    Mushrooms with
    Whipped Parsnips,
    128–129
Grilled Shrimp with Olives
    and Feta, 166
Ground Beef Casserole with
    Cheese Crust, 183
Guacamole Salad with
    Chicken, 114

H

Hawaiian Ice, 201
Herb-Marinated Cod, 162
Hobo Packets, 176
Homemade Hummus, 97
Hummus, Cheese, and
    Avocado Tostadas, 118

J

Jicama Salsa, 104

L

Lemon and Arugula Pasta,
    130–131
Lemon-Lime Detox
    Smoothie, 74
Lemon-Marinated Olives, 98
Lemon-Thyme Roasted
    Chicken, 174
Lentil-Brown Rice
    Casserole, 136

M

Marinated Bocconcini, 199
Mayonnaise, 206
Meatballs, Your Way, 182
Mexican Eggs, 87
Mint Tzatziki, 217

N

No-Cook White Sauce, 216
No-Mayo Deviled Eggs, 99
Nutty Almond Butter-
  Banana Bites, 75

P

Pesto Grilled Chicken
  Thighs, 188–189
Pico de Gallo, 212
Poached Eggs with Tomato,
  Basil, and Avocado, 88–89
Pumpkin-Sage Soup, 120

Q

Quick Curried Lentil Stew,
  122–123
Quinoa Cakes, 150–151
Quinoa "Tabbouleh,"
  142–143

R

Ratatouille, 144–145
Ratatouille-Stuffed
  Peppers, 146
Ricotta-Stuffed Spaghetti
  Squash, 134–135
Roasted Edamame with
  Cracked Pepper, 101
Roasted Eggplant
  Spread, 103

S

Savory Couch Nuts, 95
Savory Green Smoothie, 71
Scallion Tofu Dip, 102
Sesame-Ginger Soba
  Noodles, 141
Shrimp Scampi, 156–157
Simple Roasted Salmon
  with Tomatoes, 163
Slow-Cooked Creamy Black
  Beans, 117
Slow-Cooker Pot Roast, 186
Spiced Chickpeas with
  Grilled Tofu, 137–138
Spicy Roasted Chickpeas,
  92–93

Spicy Salmon Burgers, 171
Spinach and Feta Summer
  Squash "Pasta," 132–133
Spinach and White Bean
  Stew, 148–149
Spinach Salad with
  Shrimp, 170
Steak Salad with Goat
  Cheese, 112–113
Steamed Mussels with
  Saffron, 167
Strawberry Almond
  Smoothie, 73
Strawberry-Banana Cream
  Tart, 193–194
Sweet Pea Soup, 119

T

Tempeh and Swiss Chard
  Stir-Fry, 147
Turkey Meatloaf, 184

W

White Chili, 152–153

INDEX

A

Acesulfame potassium, 19
Addiction withdrawal,
    psychological effects of,
    57–58
Agave nectar, 19
Alive and Radiant Foods,
    219
Almond butter
    Nutty Almond Butter-
        Banana Bites, 75
Almond flour
    Strawberry-Banana Cream
        Tart, 193–194
"Almond Joy" Trail Mix, 202
Almond milk
    Strawberry Almond
        Smoothie, 73
Almonds, 73, 79
    "Almond Joy" Trail Mix,
        202
    Grain-Free Granola,
        79–80
    Savory Couch Nuts, 95
    Strawberry Almond
        Smoothie, 73
    The Cheese Course, 200
Amazon, 220
American Chemical
    Society, 58
*American Journal of
    Clinical Nutrition*, 26
Anchovies
    Green Goddess
        Dressing, 211
Anthocyanins, 70
Antioxidants, 71, 72, 119,
    121, 197
Applegate Farms, 219
Argentinean-Style Beef, 181
Artisana, 219

Arugula
    Arugula and White Bean
        Salad, 115
    Grilled Shrimp with
        Olives and Feta, 166
    Lemon and Arugula Pasta,
        130–131
Asiago cheese
    The Cheese Course, 200
Asian Chicken Kebabs, 185
Asian menu, 64
Asian Slaw with Thai Tofu,
    139–140
Asparagus and Prosciutto
    Salad, 116
Aspartame, 19
Au Jus, 207
Avocados, 27
    Chocolate Mousse, 192
    Cucumber Lime
        Refreshers, 197
    Green Goddess
        Dressing, 211
    Green Tea Smoothie, 72
    Guacamole Salad with
        Chicken, 114
    Hummus, Cheese, and
        Avocado Tostadas, 118
    Poached Eggs with
        Tomato, Basil, and
        Avocado, 88–89
    Savory Green Smoothie, 71

B

Bacon
    Bacon and Broccoli
        Salad, 108
    Bacon-Wrapped Chicken
        Bites, 96
    Cheesy Bacon Breakfast
        Casserole, 81–82

Creamy Spinach and
    Bacon Pie, 177
Baked Vegetable
    Chips, 105
Baked White Fish Fillets,
    158–159
Balsamic Quinoa-Spinach
    Salad, 110–111
Bananas, 27
    Banana-Walnut Morning
        "Sundae," 76
    Berry Banana Dreams, 198
    Chocolate-Almond
        Fondue, 203
    Chocolate Mousse, 192
    Lemon-Lime Detox
        Smoothie, 74
    Nutty Almond Butter-
        Banana Bites, 75
    Savory Green Smoothie, 71
    Strawberry-Banana Cream
        Tart, 193–194
Barley, 25
Basil
    Curried Carrot Soup with
        Basil, 121
    Fresh Pesto Sauce, 215
    Fresh Pickled Vegetables,
        214
    Pesto Grilled Chicken
        Thighs, 188–189
    Poached Eggs with
        Tomato, Basil, and
        Avocado, 88–89
    Ratatouille, 144–145
    Ricotta-Stuffed Spaghetti
        Squash, 134–135
    Roasted Eggplant
        Spread, 103
    Simple Roasted Salmon
        with Tomatoes, 163

Spinach and Feta Summer
Squash "Pasta," 132–133
Beans. *See* Black beans;
Cannellini beans;
Chickpeas; Pinto beans
Beef
Argentinean-Style
Beef, 181
Slow-Cooker Pot
Roast, 186
Steak Salad with Goat
Cheese, 112–113
Bell peppers
Asian Slaw with Thai
Tofu, 139–140
Chicken Fajita Lettuce
Cups, 175
Crustless Spring
Quiche, 86
Jicama Salsa, 104
Ratatouille, 144–145
Ratatouille-Stuffed
Peppers, 146
Roasted Eggplant
Spread, 103
Bergin Fruit and Nut
Company, 220
Berries, 22. *See also*
Blackberries; Blueberries;
Strawberries
Berry-Banana Dreams, 198
Berry-Coconut Cream
Parfaits, 195
Beta-carotene, 121
Beverages. *See also*
Smoothies
Chocolate Blackberry
Frappé, 70
Black Beans, Slow-Cooked
Creamy, 117
Blackberries, 22, 27
Berry-Coconut Cream
Parfaits, 195
Blackberry Shooters, 196
The Cheese Course, 200
Chocolate Blackberry
Frappé, 70

Blackened Salmon with
Cucumber Salsa,
164–165
Blood sugar, 23–24
Blueberries, 22, 27
Berry-Coconut Cream
Parfaits, 195
Blue Cheese Dressing, 210
Blue meal plan, 33
foods to avoid on, 53
meal plan, 46–47
pantry items, 49
shopping list, 48
Bocconcini
The Cheese Course, 200
Marinated Bocconcini, 199
Body, preparing for detox,
54–58
Brie
The Cheese Course, 200
British Medical Journal, 26
Broccoli, 62
Bacon and Broccoli
Salad, 108
Crustless Spring Quiche, 86
Grilled Garlic-Rosemary
Pork Tenderloin with
Steamed Broccoli,
179–180
Broth. *See* Chicken broth;
Fish stock; Vegetable
broth
Brown rice, 62
Lentil-Brown Rice
Casserole, 136
Ratatouille-Stuffed
Peppers, 146
Brunet, 113
Buckwheat, 62
Burgers. *See also*
Sandwiches
Spicy Salmon Burgers, 171
B vitamins, 136

C

Cabbage. *See* Napa cabbage
Caffeine, 25

Cannellini beans
Arugula and White Bean
Salad, 115
Spinach and White Bean
Stew, 148–149
White Chili, 152–153
Carbohydrates, 21–22
complex, 21
increasing intake of
good, 62
simple, 21
Carrots
Curried Carrot Soup with
Basil, 121
Quick Curried Lentil Stew,
122–123
Slow-Cooker Pot Roast,
186
Cauliflower, 62
Cheddar cheese
Bacon and Broccoli
Salad, 108
Cheesy Bacon Breakfast
Casserole, 81–82
Creamy Spinach and
Bacon Pie, 177
Hummus, Cheese,
and Avocado
Tostadas, 118
Lentil-Brown Rice
Casserole, 136
Mexican Eggs, 87
Cheese. *See* Asiago
cheese; Bocconcini; Brie;
Cheddar cheese; Feta
cheese; Goat cheese;
Mozzarella cheese;
Parmesan cheese;
Parmigiano-Reggiano
cheese; Pecorino Romano
cheese
Cheese Course, The, 200
Cheesy Bacon Breakfast
Casserole, 81–82
Cherry tomatoes
Simple Roasted Salmon
with Tomatoes, 163

Chia seeds
  Cucumber-Lime
    Refreshers, 197
Chicken
  Asian Chicken
    Kebabs, 185
  Bacon-Wrapped Chicken
    Bites, 96
  Chicken Fajita Lettuce
    Cups, 175
  Chicken Salad with
    Walnuts, 109
  Chicken Sausage
    Patties, 187
  Guacamole Salad with
    Chicken, 114
  Hobo Packets, 176
  Lemon-Thyme Roasted
    Chicken, 174
  Pesto Grilled Chicken
    Thighs, 188–189
Chicken broth
  Shrimp Scampi, 156–157
  Steamed Mussels with
    Saffron, 167
  White Chili, 152–153
Chickpeas
  Homemade Hummus, 97
  Spiced Chickpeas with
    Grilled Tofu, 137
  Spicy Roasted Chickpeas,
    92–93
  Spinach Salad with
    Shrimp, 170
Chile-Lime Grilled Salmon,
  160–161
Chimichurri Sauce, 213
Chocolate. See Cocoa powder
Chocolate-Almond
  Fondue, 203
Chocolate Blackberry
  Frappé, 70
Chocolate Mousse, 192
Cocaine, 57
Cocoa powder
  Chocolate-Almond
    Fondue, 203

Chocolate Blackberry
  Frappé, 70
Chocolate Mousse, 192
Coconut
  "Almond Joy" Trail
    Mix, 202
  Asian Slaw with Thai
    Tofu, 139–140
  Grain-Free Granola,
    79–80
  Quick Curried Lentil Stew,
    122–123
Coconut aminos
  Asian Chicken Kebabs, 185
  Chicken Fajita Lettuce
    Cups, 175
  Scallion Tofu Dip, 102
  Tempeh and Swiss Chard
    Stir-Fry, 147
Coconut milk
  Banana-Walnut Morning
    "Sundae," 76
  Berry-Coconut Cream
    Parfaits, 195
  Blackberry Shooters, 196
  Chocolate-Almond
    Fondue, 203
  Chocolate Blackberry
    Frappé, 70
  Chocolate Mousse, 192
  Hawaiian Ice, 201
  Pumpkin-Sage Soup, 120
  Quick Curried Lentil Stew,
    122–123
  Strawberry-Banana
    Cream Tart, 193–194
Coconut Secret, 219
Cod
  Cod and Green Beans in
    Parchment, 168–169
  Herb-Marinated Cod, 162
Complex carbohydrates, 21
Condiments
  Fresh Pickled
    Vegetables, 214
  Mayonnaise, 206
Copper, 73, 84, 115, 117

Cortisol, 24
Creamy Spinach and Bacon
  Pie, 177
Crottin de Chavignol, 113
Crunchy Kale Chips, 94
Crustless Spring Quiche, 86
Cucumbers
  Arugula and White Bean
    Salad, 115
  Asparagus and Prosciutto
    Salad, 116
  Blackened Salmon with
    Cucumber Salsa,
    164–165
  Cucumber and Tuna Salad
    Bites, 100
  Cucumber-Lime
    Refreshers, 197
  Mint Tzatziki, 217
  Quinoa "Tabbouleh,"
    142–143
  Steak Salad with Goat
    Cheese, 112–113
Curried Carrot Soup with
  Basil, 121
Curry-Ginger Pork
  Chops, 178
Cyclamate, 19

D
Daily Detox Tracker, 59
Dairy
  allowance per day, 27
Deli, 64
Detox
  after, 61–65
  Daily Detox Tracker, 59
  defined, 15
  natural sugar consumption
    and, 23–27
  preparing for, 50–59
Detox diets, 15
Dextrin, 19
Diatase, 19
Digestion, healthy, 15
Dining out, 63–64
Doctor, consulting a, 18

Dopamine, 24, 57
Double-Boiler Scrambled
    Eggs, 83
Dressings
    Blue Cheese Dressing, 210
    Green Goddess
        Dressing, 211
Dry spice rubs, 165

E

Eating habits, better, 14
Eat Wild, 220
Edamame
    Roasted Edamame with
        Cracked Pepper, 101
    Sesame-Ginger Soba
        Noodles, 141
Eden Foods, 219
Eetch, 142
Eggplant
    Eggplant Sandwiches
        with Herbed Feta,
        124–125
    Ratatouille, 144–145
    Roasted Eggplant
        Spread, 103
Eggs
    Cheesy Bacon Breakfast
        Casserole, 81–82
    Creamy Spinach and
        Bacon Pie, 177
    Crustless Spring
        Quiche, 86
    Double-Broiler Scrambled
        Eggs, 83
    Egg and Prosciutto-
        Stuffed Mushroom
        Caps, 84–85
    Mexican Eggs, 87
    No-Mayo Deviled
        Eggs, 99
    Poached Eggs with
        Tomato, Basil, and
        Avocado, 88–89
    Quinoa Cakes, 150–151
Egg yolks
    Mayonnaise, 206

Endocannabinoids, 58
Endorphins, 58
Erythritol, 19
Ethyl maltol, 19
Exercise, 17, 58

F

Fennel
    Baked Vegetable Chips,
        105
    Steamed Mussels with
        Saffron, 167
Feta cheese
    Eggplant Sandwiches with
        Herbed Feta, 124–125
    Grilled Shrimp with
        Olives and Feta, 166
    Ratatouille, 144–145
    Spinach and Feta Summer
        Squash "Pasta,"
        132–133
    Spinach and White Bean
        Stew, 148–149
Fiber, 21, 27, 117, 119
Fish. See Seafood and fish
Fish stock
    Steamed Mussels with
        Saffron, 167
Flaxseed
    Chocolate Blackberry
        Frappé, 70
    Grain-Free Granola, 79–80
    Strawberry-Almond
        Smoothie, 73
Flour. See Almond flour
Folate, 117
Food Allergy Research and
    Education (FARE), 26–27
Foods, avoiding, 52
    on Blue plan, 53
    on Green plan, 53
    on Orange plan, 53
Frappé, Chocolate
    Blackberry, 70
Fresh Pesto Sauce, 215
Fresh Pickled
    Vegetables, 214

Fresh Tomato Sauce,
    208–209
    Ricotta-Stuffed Spaghetti
        Squash, 134–135
Fructamyl, 19
Fruit, allowance per day, 27.
    See also specific

G

Garbanzo beans. See
    Chickpeas
Garrotxa, 113
Ginger
    Tempeh and Swiss Chard
        Stir-Fry, 147
Gliadin, 25
Gluten, 25
Gluten-free diet, 25
Glutenin, 25
Glycerol, 19
Glycyrrhizin, 19
Goat cheese
    buying, 113
    Steak Salad with Goat
        Cheese, 112–113
Grain-Free Granola, 79–80
Grains, 25–26
Greek yogurt
    Berry Banana Dreams, 198
    Blue Cheese Dressing, 210
    Breakfast Grains with
        Hazelnuts, 77–78
    Chicken Salad with
        Walnuts, 109
    Mint Tzatziki, 217
Green beans, 62
    Cod and Green Beans in
        Parchment, 168–169
Green Goddess Dressing,
    96, 211
    Steak Salad with Goat
        Cheese, 112–113
Green meal plan, 32
    foods to avoid on, 53
    meal plan, 42–43
    pantry items, 45
    shopping list, 44

Green Tea Smoothie, 72
Grilled Garlic-Rosemary
    Pork Tenderloin with
    Steamed Broccoli, 179–180
Grilled Portobello
    Mushrooms with
    Whipped Parsnips,
    128–129
Grilled Shrimp with Olives
    and Feta, 166
Grocery bill, 16
Ground beef
    Ground Beef Casserole
        with Cheese Crust, 183
    Meatballs, Your Way, 182
Guacamole Salad with
    Chicken, 114

H
Haddock
    Baked White Fish Fillets,
        158–159
Ham. See Prosciutto
Hawaiian Ice, 201
Hazelnuts
    Breakfast Grains with
        Hazelnuts, 77–78
    Grain-Free Granola, 79–80
Healthier lifestyle,
    beginning a, 13–14
Hearts of palm
    Steak Salad with Goat
        Cheese, 112–113
Herb-Marinated Cod, 162
Hobo Packets, 176
Hoebel, Bart, 24
Hummus
    Homemade Hummus, 97
    Hummus, Cheese, and
        Avocado Tostadas, 118
Hunger, 64
Hydrogenated starch
    hydrolysate, 19

I
Insulin, role of, 23–24
Iron, 79, 119, 130

Isomalt, 19
Italian menu, 64

J
Jalapeño peppers
    Mexican Eggs, 87
    Pico de Gallo, 212
    Roasted Eggplant
        Spread, 103
Jicama Salsa, 104
Journaling, 55–56

K
Kale
    Crunchy Kale Chips, 94
    Lemon-Lime Detox
        Smoothie, 74
    Savory Green Smoothie, 71
Kebabs, Asian Chicken, 185
King Arthur Flour, 220
Kisir, 142
Kitchen
    preparing, for detox diet,
        51–54
    time spent in, 16–17

L
Lactitol, 19
Lactose, 26
    disease issues related
        to, 15
Lactose intolerance, 26
Lectins, 26
Legumes, 26. See also
    Chickpeas
Lemon-Marinated Olives, 98
    Spinach Salad with
        Shrimp, 170
    The Cheese Course, 200
Lemons, 22, 27
    getting juice from, 74
    Lemon and Arugula Pasta,
        130–131
    Lemon-Lime Detox
        Smoothie, 74
    Lemon-Marinated
        Olives, 98

Lemon-Thyme Roasted
    Chicken, 174
Lentils
    Lentil-Brown Rice
        Casserole, 136
    Quick Curried Lentil Stew,
        122–123
Lettuce. See also Mixed
    greens
    Chicken Fajita Lettuce
        Cups, 175
    Spicy Salmon Burgers, 171
Limes, 22, 27
    getting juice from, 74
    Lemon-Lime Detox
        Smoothie, 74
Low calorie foods, 28
Low-density lipoprotein, 23
Lutein, 71

M
Maltitol, 19
Maltodextrin, 19
Manganese, 73, 117, 136
Mannitol, 19
Marinated Bocconcini, 199
Mayo Clinic, 26
Mayonnaise, 206
    Bacon and Broccoli
        Salad, 108
    Blue Cheese Dressing, 210
    Cucumber and Tuna Salad
        Bites, 100
    Green Goddess
        Dressing, 211
    No-Cook White Sauce, 216
Measurement conversions,
    221
Meatballs, Your Way, 182
Meatloaf
    Turkey Meatloaf, 184
Menu items, sugar in
    common, 64–65
Mexican Eggs, 87
Milk. See also Almond milk;
    Coconut milk
    allergies to, 27

Mint Tzatziki, 217
Mixed greens
  Asparagus and Prosciutto
    Salad, 116
  Guacamole Salad with
    Chicken, 114
  Quinoa Cakes, 150–151
Molybdenum, 117, 136
Morphine, 57
Mozzarella cheese
  Ratatouille-Stuffed
    Peppers, 146
Mushrooms, 62
  Egg and Prosciutto-
    Stuffed Mushroom
    Caps, 84–85
  Grilled Portobello
    Mushrooms with
    Whipped Parsnips,
    128–129
  Spinach and Feta Summer
    Squash "Pasta,"
    132–133
Mussels, Steamed, with
  Saffron, 167

N
Nachos, 114
Napa cabbage
  Asian Slaw with Thai
    Tofu, 139–140
National Institute of
  Diabetes and Digestive
  and Kidney Diseases, 15
Natural sugar, 21–22
  detox and, 23–27
Neotame, 19
Nestle, Marion, 64
Nicotine, 57
No-Cook White Sauce, 216
No-Mayo Deviled
  Eggs, 99
Nuts. See Almonds;
  Hazelnuts; Pecans;
  Pistachios; Walnuts
Nutty Almond Butter-
  Banana Bites, 75

O
Olives
  Grilled Shrimp with
    Olives and Feta, 166
  Lemon-Marinated
    Olives, 98
Omega-3 fatty acids, 79
Once Again, 219
Onions
  Chicken Fajita Lettuce
    Cups, 175
  Fresh Tomato Sauce,
    208–209
  Ratatouille, 144–145
  Spiced Chickpeas with
    Grilled Tofu, 137
  Spinach and White Bean
    Stew, 148–149
  White Chili, 152–153
Orange meal plan, 31–32
  foods to avoid on, 53
  meal plan, 34–35
  pantry items, 37
  shopping list, 36

P
Panocha, 19
Pantry items
  for Blue meal plan, 49
  for Green meal plan, 45
  for Orange meal plan, 37
  for Yellow meal plan, 41
Parchment
  Cod and Green Beans in
    Parchment, 168–169
Parmesan cheese
  Asparagus and Prosciutto
    Salad, 116
  Ground Beef Casserole
    with Cheese Crust, 183
  Ricotta-Stuffed Spaghetti
    Squash, 134–135
Parmigiano-Reggiano
  cheese
  Fresh Pesto Sauce, 215
Parsley
  Chimichurri Sauce, 213

Parsnips
  Baked Vegetable Chips,
    105
  Grilled Portobello Mush-
    rooms with Whipped
    Parsnips, 128–129
Pasta, Lemon and Arugula,
  130–131
Peas
  Sweet Pea Soup, 119
Pecans
  Grain-Free Granola, 79–80
  Savory Couch Nuts, 95
Pecorino Romano cheese
  Ground Beef Casserole
    with Cheese Crust, 183
  Meatballs, Your Way, 182
Penzey's Spices, 219
Pesto Grilled Chicken
  Thighs, 188–189
Phosphatidylserine, 148
Phosphorus, 136
Phytoestrogens, 70
Pico de Gallo, 212
Pine nuts
  Fresh Pesto Sauce, 215
  Pesto Grilled Chicken
    Thighs, 188–189
Pinto beans
  White Chili, 152–153
Pistachios
  Savory Couch Nuts, 95
Pizza, 65
Poached Eggs with Tomato,
  Basil, and Avocado,
  88–89
Poaching, adding vinegar
  to water for, 88
Poblano pepper
  White Chili, 152–153
Polyacetylene, 128
Polydextrose, 19
Pork. See also Prosciutto
  Creamy Spinach and
    Bacon Pie, 177
  Curry-Ginger Pork
    Chops, 178

Grilled Garlic-Rosemary
    Pork Tenderloin with
    Steamed Broccoli,
    179–180
Potassium, 84, 115
Princeton Neuroscience
    Institute, 24
Prosciutto
    Asparagus and Prosciutto
        Salad, 116
    Egg and Prosciutto-
        Stuffed Mushroom
        Caps, 84–85
Proteins, 118, 119
    fighting cravings
        with, 62
Psychological effects of
    addiction withdrawal,
    57–58
Psychopharmacology, 58
Pumpkin-Sage Soup, 120
Pumpkin seeds
    Bacon and Broccoli
        Salad, 108
    Balsamic Quinoa-Spinach
        Salad, 110–111
    Grain-Free Granola, 79–80
    Steak Salad with Goat
        Cheese, 112–113

Q
Quiche, Crustless Spring, 86
Quinoa
    Balsamic Quinoa-Spinach
        Salad, 110–111
    Breakfast Grains with
        Hazelnuts, 77–78
    Quinoa Cakes, 150–151
    Quinoa "Tabbouleh,"
        142–143

R
Ratatouille, 144–145
    Ratatouille-Stuffed
        Peppers, 146
Refined sugar, 22
Resources, 219–220

Ricotta-Stuffed Spaghetti
    Squash, 134–135
Roasted Edamame with
    Cracked Pepper, 101
Roasted Eggplant Spread, 103
Roasted red peppers
    Ground Beef Casserole
        with Cheese Crust, 183
Rocket. *See* Arugula
Romaine lettuce
    Steak Salad with Goat
        Cheese, 112–113
Rosemary
    Grilled Garlic-Rosemary
        Pork Tenderloin with
        Steamed Broccoli,
        179–180
Rye, 25

S
Saccharin, 19
Saffron
    Steamed Mussels with
        Saffron, 167
Sage
    Pumpkin-Sage Soup, 120
Salads, 64. *See also* Dressings
    Arugula and White Bean
        Salad, 115
    Asparagus and Prosciutto
        Salad, 116
    Bacon and Broccoli
        Salad, 108
    Balsamic Quinoa-Spinach
        Salad, 110–111
    Chicken Salad with
        Walnuts, 109
    Guacamole Salad with
        Chicken, 114
    Spinach Salad with
        Shrimp, 170
    Steak Salad with Goat
        Cheese, 112–113
Salmon
    Blackened Salmon with
        Cucumber Salsa,
        164–165

Chile-Lime Grilled
    Salmon, 160–161
Simple Roasted Salmon
    with Tomatoes, 163
Spicy Salmon Burgers, 171
Sandwiches. *See also*
    Burgers
    Eggplant Sandwiches with
        Herbed Feta, 124–125
Sauces
    Au Jus, 207
    Chimichurri Sauce, 213
    Fresh Pesto Sauce, 215
    Fresh Tomato Sauce,
        208–209
    Mint Tzatziki, 217
    No-Cook White Sauce, 216
    Pico de Gallo, 212
Savory Couch Nuts, 95
Savory Green Smoothie, 71
Scallions
    Asian Slaw with Thai
        Tofu, 139–140
    Scallion Tofu Dip, 102
Seafood and fish, 155–171
    Baked White Fish Fillets,
        158–159
    Blackened Salmon with
        Cucumber Salsa,
        164–165
    Chile-Lime Grilled
        Salmon, 160–161
    Cod and Green Beans in
        Parchment, 168–169
    Cucumber and Tuna Salad
        Bites, 100
    Grilled Shrimp with
        Olives and Feta, 166
    Herb-Marinated Cod, 162
    Shrimp Scampi, 156–157
    Simple Roasted Salmon
        with Tomatoes, 163
    Spicy Salmon Burgers, 171
    Spinach Salad with
        Shrimp, 170
    Steamed Mussels with
        Saffron, 167

Seeds. *See* Chia seeds; Flaxseed; Pumpkin seeds; Sunflower seeds
Selenium, 79
Sesame-Ginger Soba Noodles, 141
Shopping list
  for Blue meal plan, 48
  for Green meal plan, 44
  for Orange meal plan, 36
  for Yellow meal plan, 40
Shrimp
  Grilled Shrimp with Olives and Feta, 166
  Shrimp Scampi, 156–157
  Spinach Salad with Shrimp, 170
Sides
  Hummus, Cheese, and Avocado Tostadas, 118
  Slow-Cooked Creamy Black Beans, 117
Silk, 219
Simple carbohydrates, 21
Simple Roasted Salmon with Tomatoes, 163
Simply Organics, 219
Slaw, Asian, wth Thai Tofu, 139–140
Sleep, 62–63
  better, 14–15
Slow-Cooked Creamy Black Beans, 117
Slow-Cooker Pot Roast, 186
Smoothies
  Green Tea Smoothie, 72
  Lemon-Lime Detox Smoothie, 74
  Savory Green Smoothie, 71
  Strawberry Almond Smoothie, 73
Snacks, 90–105
  Bacon-Wrapped Chicken Bites, 96
  Baked Vegetable Chips, 105

Crunchy Kale Chips, 94
Cucumber and Tuna Salad Bites, 100
Homemade Hummus, 97
Jicama Salsa, 104
Lemon-Marinated Olives, 98
No-Mayo Deviled Eggs, 99
Roasted Edamame with Cracked Pepper, 101
Roasted Eggplant Spread, 103
Savory Couch Nuts, 95
Scallion Tofu Dip, 102
Spicy Roasted Chickpeas, 92–93
Soba noodles, 141
  Sesame-Ginger Soba Noodles, 141
Sorbitol, 19
Soups
  Curried Carrot Soup with Basil, 121
  Pumpkin-Sage Soup, 120
  Sweet Pea Soup, 119
Spaghetti squash
  Ricotta-Stuffed Spaghetti Squash, 134–135
Spiced Chickpeas with Grilled Tofu, 137–138
Spicy Roasted Chickpeas, 92–93
Spicy Salmon Burgers, 171
Spinach
  Baked White Fish Fillets, 158–159
  Balsamic Quinoa-Spinach Salad, 110–111
  Creamy Spinach and Bacon Pie, 177
  Green Tea Smoothie, 72
  Ratatouille, 144–145
  Ricotta-Stuffed Spaghetti Squash, 134–135
  Savory Green Smoothie, 71

Scallion Tofu Dip, 102
Spiced Chickpeas with Grilled Tofu, 137
Spinach and Feta Summer Squash "Pasta," 132–133
Spinach and White Bean Stew, 148–149
Spinach Salad with Shrimp, 170
Squash. *See* Spaghetti squash; Winter squash; Yellow squash
Starch, 21
Steak Salad with Goat Cheese, 112–113
Steamed Mussels with Saffron, 167
Stew
  Quick Curried Lentil Stew, 122–123
  Spinach and White Bean Stew, 148–149
Stir Fry
  Tempeh and Swiss Chard Stir-Fry, 147
Strawberries, 27, 73
  Berry-Coconut Cream Parfaits, 195
  Chocolate-Almond Fondue, 203
  Strawberry Almond Smoothie, 73
  Strawberry-Banana Cream Tart, 193–194
Sucrose, 21
Sucralose, 19
Sugar
  addiction to, 24
  in common menu items, 64–65
  consumption of, 9
  natural, 21–22
  other names for, 19
  readiness to quit, 13–18
  refined, 22
  reintroducing into diet, 63

Sugar bingeing, 57
Sugar-free foods, 28
Sugar-free, staying, 61–63
Sugar overload, 22–23
Sugar withdrawal, 17
Sunflower seeds
  Bacon and Broccoli
    Salad, 108
  Grain-Free Granola, 79–80
Sweet Pea Soup, 119
Sweet potatoes
  Baked Vegetable
    Chips, 105
  Quinoa Cakes, 150–151
Swiss chard
  Tempeh and Swiss Chard
    Stir-Fry, 147

T
Tabbouleh
  Quinoa "Tabbouleh,"
    142–143
Tagatose, 19
Tahini
  Homemade Hummus, 97
Tamari
  Scallion Tofu Dip, 102
  Sesame-Ginger Soba
    Noodles, 141
Tempeh and Swiss Chard
  Stir-Fry, 147
10-Day Sugar Detox, 6–7, 9
  duration of, 18
  expectations during,
    16–17
  pantry items, 49
  reasons to do a, 14–15
  shopping list, 48
Thai Kitchen, 219
Tilapia
  Baked White Fish
    Fillets, 158–159
Today's Dietitian, 24
Tofu
  Asian Slaw with Thai
    Tofu, 139–140
  Scallion Tofu Dip, 102

Spiced Chickpeas with
  Grilled Tofu, 137
Tomatillos
  White Chili, 152–153
Tomatoes, 27. See also
  Cherry tomatoes
  Balsamic Quinoa-Spinach
    Salad, 110–111
  Fresh Tomato Sauce,
    208–209
  Guacamole Salad with
    Chicken, 114
  Lemon and Arugula Pasta,
    130–131
  Mexican Eggs, 87
  Pico de Gallo, 212
  Poached Eggs with
    Tomato, Basil, and
    Avocado, 88–89
  Quinoa "Tabbouleh,"
    142–143
  Ratatouille, 144–145
  Savory Green
    Smoothie, 71
  Slow-Cooker Pot Roast, 186
  Spinach and Feta Summer
    Squash "Pasta," 132–133
  Spinach and White Bean
    Stew, 148–149
Tortillas
  Hummus, Cheese, and
    Avocado Tostadas, 118
Toxins, 15
Treacle, 19
Tuna, Cucumber and, Salad
  Bites, 100
Turkey Meatloaf, 184
Type 2 diabetes, 23

U
U.S. Wellness Meats, 219

V
The Vegan Store, 220
Vegetable broth
  Balsamic Quinoa-Spinach
    Salad, 110–111

Curried Carrot Soup with
  Basil, 121
Pumpkin-Sage Soup, 120
Shrimp Scampi, 156–157
Spiced Chickpeas with
  Grilled Tofu, 137
Sweet Pea Soup, 119
White Chili, 152–153
Vegetables, Fresh
  Pickled, 214
Vinegar, adding to water for
  poaching, 88
Vitamin A, 115, 116, 130
Vitamin C, 70, 71, 115, 116, 130
Vitamin E, 73, 79, 116, 203
Vitamin K, 115, 116, 130

W
Walnuts
  Banana-Walnut Morning
    "Sundae," 76
  Chicken Salad with
    Walnuts, 109
  Grain-Free Granola,
    79–80
  Nutty Almond Butter-
    Banana Bites, 75
  Savory Couch Nuts, 95
Water, 64
WebMD, 26
Weight loss, 14
Wheat, 25
White Chili, 152–153
Whole-grain pasta, 62
Winter squash, 120
Worcestershire sauce
  Savory Couch Nuts, 95

X
Xylitol, 19

Y
Yellow meal plan, 32
  meal plan, 38–39
  pantry items, 41
Yellow squash
  Ratatouille, 144–145

Spinach and Feta Summer
    Squash "Pasta,"
    132–133
Yogurt. *See* Greek yogurt

Z

Zeaxanthin, 71
Zero calorie foods, 28
Zucchini, 62
    Spinach and Feta Summer
        Squash "Pasta,"
        132–133

CPSIA information can be obtained
at www.ICGtesting.com
Printed in the USA
LVHW05s0422280418
574919LV00001B/1/P

9 781623 154264